Group Analysis for Refugees Experiencing Trauma

In this prescient and sensitive volume, Aida Alayarian looks at how psychoanalysis in group settings can benefit refugees and others who have experienced trauma, with an express focus on transference and countertransference.

Group Analysis for Refugees Experiencing Trauma offers a comprehensive overview of trauma from a psychoanalytic perspective, before delving into the nuance of trauma experienced by asylum seekers, refugees and those who have gone through other forms of human rights violations. Through clinical vignettes, Alayarian highlights the importance of the resilience that can be brought about from group sessions and shared experience in helping to heal the wounds of trauma. She looks at the vital role of social injustice and shows how this can be directly applied to work with other groups experiencing human rights violations, destitution, and loss. She shows how looking at relational patterns as a means of understanding conscious, unconscious, and subconscious thought processes can provide essential breakthroughs with patients, as well as the importance of paying close attention to countertransference to avoid a breakdown of the clinical relationship.

Using psychoanalytic theories from intercultural perspectives to show the multidimensional nature of work with patients, this book is essential reading for psychoanalysts, psychologists, psychiatrists, and other mental health experts working with refugees and patients experiencing trauma.

Aida Alayarian is a psychoanalyst working in the UK. She is the co-founder, former clinical director and CEO, and current chair of trustees of the Refugee Therapy Centre, a charity in north London. She is the author of *Resilience, Suffering and Creativity* (2007), *Consequences of Denial: The Armenian Genocide* (2008), *Trauma, Torture and Dissociation: A Psychoanalytic View* (2011), *Handbook of Working with Children, Trauma, and Resilience: An Intercultural Psychoanalytic View* (2015) and *Children of Refugees: Torture, Human Rights, and Psychological Consequences* (2016).

Group Analysis for Refugees Experiencing Trauma

Aida Alayarian

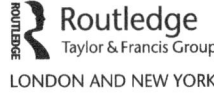
Routledge
Taylor & Francis Group

LONDON AND NEW YORK

Designed cover image: 501room/Getty Images

First published 2024
by Routledge
4 Park Square, Milton Park, Abingdon, Oxon OX14 4RN

and by Routledge
605 Third Avenue, New York, NY 10158

Routledge is an imprint of the Taylor & Francis Group, an informa business

British Library Cataloguing in Publication Data
A catalogue record for this book is available from the British Library

ISBN: 9781032512433 (hbk)
ISBN: 9781032512402 (pbk)
ISBN: 9781003401322 (ebk)

DOI: 10.4324/9781003401322

Typeset in Times New Roman
by Taylor & Francis Books

Contents

Introduction

In this book I will be looking at psychoanalytical theory and its clincial implications. I also will address the psychiatric medical model of post-traumatic stress disorder (PTSD) and characteristics that can commonly relate with trauma. Working with refugees and others who have endured trauma, whether individually or in the group setting, I think post-traumatic stress is the normal reaction to the abnormal situation, and I prefer not to address it as a disorder. I refer to *symptoms* rather than disorder.

I address the concept of self and the importance of intercultural relations between patients and analysts to enable more psychic space in which people can talk to themselves internally to regulate pain, and to protect themselves from too many vulnerable feelings. This unbreakable part of the self, safe-guards a traumatised person from collapsing emotionally when the external world is dangerous, unpredictable, overpowering and life-threatening. I shall discuss the creation of the false self that may be presented by patients as a construct to hide and protect the true self from what feels a life-threatening danger. In some people with good enough early development, a false self may have been developed as a defence mechanism to survive atrocity. Having said this, in such characteristics the person function is not based on the real self. In an attuned false self-organisation, patients who presents an amenable, submissive, compliant and polite attitude may be seeking approval based on the thinking this is a socially accepted manner. So, the tendency towards falseness for the person serves to allow relation, interpersonal involvement and acceptance in the new environment.

I present the importance of the assessment or the first interview as the most significant juncture in the patient–therapist relationship and also to decide whether group can be beneficial. The patient experience of feeling of having a listened other may be quite unique, and a profoundly positive and idealising relationship may develop. One of the important areas in assess-ment is making enquiries to recognise patients Oedipal or pre-Oedipal, looking for strengths of ego, self or drive, indeed patients' vulnerability and resiliency, and the type of dissociation used as defence. In the process of assessments for each group I will be considering potential participants'

DOI: 10.4324/9781003401322-1

language, age, race, gender, ethnicity, social and economic class, sexuality and sexual orientation; and focusing on participants level of resiliency, while exploring vulnerability as a necessary component of the capacity to exercise the participants traumatic experience; consider the interplay between tradition, risk-taking, vulnerability, strength and creativity, considering associations of individual to their early childhood developments to their current cultural, political and economic contexts; to their personal and professional life and the development of the established order each were familiars with and how group can provide possibilities to grew and transform to their desire, for example hope of where to work soon and what can facilitate this.

In each chapter, with brief vignettes I highlight how a group provided me with great learning opportunities that at times felt too challenging in the midst of work, and at times induced stress for me, especially when I with other members of the group faced with an acute crisis of a group member that was beyond the group work, therefore in countertransference I had to deal with extreme feelings of helplessness, as well as group difference transference. This was specifically challenging when issues were external and beyond the group (i.e. immigration refusals, disbursing, court hearings, homelessness, and lack of any finance after refusal), and therefore attendance may not advisable under such circumstances.

An outstanding factor in the beneficial results of psychoanalytic group therapy is the multitude and variety of the interrelationships that take place in groups. The transference and countertransference's are different from individual analysis where a person sees the analyst individually and react just to one person and projects all the emotional prototypes repetitions formed and inaugurated in childhood to the analyst in transference. The occurrence and identification of these patterns and reactions are a most important factor in an improved and enriched outcome of analytic process strengthening patients' personality and psychological health. For that reason, although individual therapy alone can be successful compared to group analysis might be restrictive, since it cannot arouse the whole range of deep emotions towards different individuals in one setting. In group the different personalities of the participants can evoke a variety of differentiated emotional reactions from each individual to a number of personalities within the group and by doing so become aware and identify specific feelings, behaviour prototypes, tensions and conflicts.

In the individual work the analyst is limited by the patient's subjectively coloured reports of unpleasant incident and demonstrative reactions to them. In contrast in the group interventions, the analyst and the group can noticeably and objectively identify and distinguish the behaviour in which each person's protective deafens and emotional patterns alter perception of reality. Consequently, the group members gradually will accomplish insight into own divergences and deviances from objectivity. People who have undesirable personality traits and conduct prototypes can benefit much more in the group than in individual analysis. This is because the psychoanalyst is only one person in pointing out such weaknesses or shortcomings to the patient by interpretations, and in doing so, always have to be mindful not to offend the patients and harm the therapeutic relationship, but through group interactions and other participants in the group will more freely point imperfections or mistakes to each other. In some ways the group setting and interactions between members is more like the outer world we live in as contrasted with the shielded fortification that analyst may adopt in individual sessions.

Many patients initially in the process of assessments, when I suggested joining group, they object to the idea and thought it is in no way they can talk about their experiences in present of other people, either because they feel uncomfortable to talk speak about their problems and also because of fear of other people from their community and lack of trust. Of course, such fears and mistrust are indeed connected to the trauma they have endured, acknowledging this with individual concern was helpful and beneficial as the right strategy to work through fears and mistrust rather than avoid addressing them. I will tell such patients, come for 6 weeks and try, you can talk about anything you feel comfortable or stay silence if you so wish. On this condition they agreed to join the group and practically more or less these fears and lack of trust lessen and gradually diminished after a few sessions being in the group, in some cases from the first session.

Some people have the inaccurate impression that the reason for group analysis is because it is less expensive compared to individual psychoanalytic treatments. Although the group work might be more cost effective than individual, but it is not the reason for forming a group. The success of therapeutic interventions very much depends on the degree to which patients repressed emotions are stimulated, transported to consciousness, communicated in an articulated manner and worked through. This process often stimulates considerably in group interactions than individual analysis and can result into important areas of emotional disturbance that might not otherwise been identified at conscious level. Group provides an opportunity for participants to express thoughts and feelings. Some people may participate actively from the beginning and others may choose to remain silent for a while. Whichever preference patients may have, following others during the sessions will be helpful to gain awareness expressing feelings and thoughts throughout the meetings even in cases that people have difficulty in verbalising feelings. So, for many people who may stay silence the first stage in the group is listening and learning to identify and name feelings and come out of confusion that are more often than not mere defences against and rationalisations of real feelings.

The aim of this book is to demonstrate the psychoanalytic knowledge and methods specifically within group therapy, expressly focusing on treatments for people who have endured trauma; examining the transference and countertransference. Whether we are working with children, adults, parents or couples both individually or in group, an essential therapeutic purpose is to enable and enhance the patients' competence for emotional adjustment and decree, providing psychological tools helping them effectively identify and understand their emotions, so that they are able to process and respond and express them safely. Before our patients can learn to self-regulate, we need to achieve co-regulation, which is foundation to affecting regulation to process emotion, especially if the person surrounded by other traumatised people.

As this book is about trauma, with specific reference to refugees as a group who are traumatised. Understanding trauma is a central for both a practical (vignettes and case studies) and theoretical (psychoanalysis) challenge. Psychoanalytical group work will mainly be from a relational perspective, with focus on resilience and vulnerability and the view that childhood trauma of refugee patient endured atrocity in adult due to the socio-political milieu is a dual narration. My therapeutic method is based on psychoanalytic theory of group work with specific focus on intercultural approach to what happens in family, groups and organisations. It combines a theoretical approach to understanding family dynamics and other group and to identify power dynamics at play be it ethnic gender or other issues and to use psychoanalytic ideas to understand the relation between their experiences, the expression of feeling with the group. The emphasis will be on the unconscious processes that I observe in groups, the processes which are typically overlooked by the therapeutic intervention and study on refugees as the focus will be on other aspects.

In other chapters, I will address discourse about trauma in general, and from psychoanalytical theory and trauma of refugees specifically. A chapter will focus on group and psychoanalytic theory on group. I shall briefly also examine the paradoxes of psychoanalysis, focusing on the unique subjectivity of the analyst and patient that is inherent in psychoanalytic practice, and the attention given necessarily to complex and ambiguous material. Despite briefly addressing element of paradox, as knowledge is always subject to refutation and profoundly influenced by subjective views of reality and relativity at that particular moment, I argue that psychoanalysis still satisfies the parameters of clinical practice, and specifically within intercultural context. I then will be designating a chapter to transference and important of countertransference. I will look at the theory of trauma in general and childhood trauma from psychoanalytic perspectives and external trauma in adult life due to the human right violations and impunity. Throughout the chapters to support the theory and discussions, I shall present brief vignettes.

Looking back, I realise that it is over three decades since I established the first group in the UK within the NHS and other charity and children's services, and later (since 1999) at the Refugee Therapy Centre. I feel both joy and sadness when I contemplate the progress, the changes and the many positive and negative influences experienced during the course of time on patients and me. The therapeutic intervention for people who endured and affected by trauma is developing as the world is a relentlessly changing environment in its physical, technological, power, politics and human dimensions. The velocity of change is increased by the ongoing reduction of resources in financing public service and within this book subject the therapeutic intervention. The search for funding and the search for new approaches, becoming one of the priority and the main restorative needs for human right services to keep the limited resources to be used best to serve those in needs. As a clinician working with the most traumatised people as the result of war, torture and other human rights violations, it is vital to think and reflect: how can we work effectively under such conditions we are exposed to in the new world? How can we challenge what we take to be the standards and medians for a healthy organisational life? How can we find space to think objectively while under pressure, and discover the potential for creative engagement with others in our separate and joint tasks, focusing to recognise and value our differences and commonalities. The purpose of this book is therefore to identify and denote opportunities find in the group work over thirty years focusing of resiliency and pattern of attachments for understanding conscious, subconscious and unconscious processes, rational and irrational, that analysts can assist patients in working with individuals or groups. With this in mind, we learn how to constantly observe, assess, reassess and analyse conscious and unconscious processes of group dynamics. I particularly pay attention to countertransference as a significant therapeutic encounter, which is often overlooked or not adequately recognised. This does not mean that as professionals, we do not face challenges within clinical practice working with patients who have endured torture, violence or other extreme human rights violations. Minimising the role of such countertransference has the potential to not only act as a destructive force potentially leading to breakdown for the clinicians, but also undermine the progress toward increased resiliency available to the patients through the therapeutic encounter. From a psychoanalytic and philosophical theories and view, this book will explore the multidimensional nature of working with people endured trauma, countertransference from both practical and theoretical perspectives, examining the impact on clinical discipline, therapist/patient relations and psychological health for both. By recognising the invariable potential for harmful and disadvantageous consequences of countertransference, it is up to us, as therapists, to monitor and help ourselves in order to ethically fulfil our role of serving those we set ourselves to help. In order for a patient to move beyond a restrictive view of relationships, their emotions and transference must be constantly acknowledged, interpreted and analysed; in much the same way, as therapists countertransference as both party are faced with the same challenge, and must give equal attention to this relational reaction in the therapeutic process. Drawing on classical and contemporary psychoanalytic theory, and its philosopher critiques, throughout the book, I will argue that transference and countertransference has both a useful and injurious capacity, offering a window of insight into the self and others while threatening to unhinge the constructive nature of the therapeutic encounter, and thus our ethical obligation, if, left unattended. Analysing ourselves and our countertransferences, in supervision and or other self-reflective practice, is the correct way in which we can ensure our commitment to ethical clinical practice which consists the true ethos of psychoanalysis.

I will look at ways in which certainties and uncertainties of individuals within groups may paralyse the thinking and be transferred to others; this at times may help group members to learn how groups jointly can work and construct a reality that despite the fact that considered external from all group members apart from one, within group dynamics learning and what seem to be unchangeable may turn to be changeable for transformation; I will be exploring rational and irrational encounters presented in group settings, and carry out trials to look at ways of engaging with difference within intercultural settings.

Chapter 1

Refugee Therapy Centre

The Refugee Therapy Centre (RTC) is an intercultural psychoanalytic therapy centre for provision of services. It initially started with psychoanalytic psychotherapy for traumatised refugees, unconditionally based on their needs. We grew from a small group of enthusiastic idealists, dreaming of making a difference in this world in a small room, to one of the leading organisations in this field in a large Victorian building with more than fifteen consulting rooms, offices, board, training and conference rooms. Year after year, members of staff, with their tremendous dedication, allowed the Centre to thrive even against many difficulties in the climate of political changes and financial difficulties. In the past the work of the RTC has been supported by over 90 volunteer psychotherapists, supervisors and medical students as mentors continuously endeavouring to cultivate a caring community within the Centre while providing the foundational services that are essential to meeting the needs of the people who come to the Centre for help. I feel grateful to all those who so full-heartedly join us to support the centre's work, making a strong team, in combination with the generous support for a promising future. The significant commitment of professionals providing to serve children, young people and their families with humility and so gracefully down to earth and without complaint. I trust these kinds of commitments are rare to achieve and I feel privileged to be able to work with and have responsibility to lead and learned from such a wonderful team for many years. I sincerely appreciate their outstanding work and for every day I learn from my colleagues how not to lose sight of people's needs and the best way of serving them and bringing human rights aspect of our work to life for those we seek to serve.

It goes without saying that for a charity like the RTC there are always serious financial challenges in the climate where healthcare organisations are operating. I personally am proud of our successful struggle to keep high standards in teaching, training, clinical work and research and to continue to provide therapy, practical support and mentorship to those in needs. In the world we are living sadly we are far from provision of ideal services that we set ourselves to provide. Thinking about the explosive situation in the world

DOI: 10.4324/9781003401322-2

and specifically in Middle East, in Africa, the humanitarian crisis in the Mediterranean, the wide-spreading phenomenon of religious radicalisation, the features of the political debate around those issues, the recent response of the people and people entitled to vote the future seems to be bleak. Despite these, we increased academic activities and partnerships with universities, mainly with East London University, the Department of Psychology Master programme in Psychoanalytic Psychotherapy with Queen Mary University of London, and Department of Psychiatry for a Professional Doctorate in Intercultural Psychoanalytic Psychotherapy.

From the clinical point of view, one of the important achievements was start of innovative groups for LGBTs (the first in the UK) and a separate men's group. This highlights one of the greatest qualities of the Centre. The outstanding creativity of the therapists and their absolute lack of fear of innovation, something which always runs the risk of being labelled unorthodox in the psychoanalytic field, those were continuity on the path of the learning from our patients, adjusting theories and practices to the characteristics of the intercultural gap between Western theories and non-Western cultures. The staff of the Centre with motivation continued to be willing to make a difference in the lives of patients, based on the ethical ideas and stance that a better world is always possible if we want it. As a result the Centre responds to hardship in its own resilience, motivation, strength, innovation and creativity, i.e. the principles and the human qualities on which we base all treatments to our patients, indeed the qualities we have learnt from them all.

The Centre's remit is:

- Helping refugees feel empowered to deal with their psychological distress by offering a culturally and linguistically sensitive therapeutic service. Providing supportive and containing environment in which people who have endured trauma are better able to understand their feelings and experiences.
- Helping to ease the demanding and intricate processes of adaptation many refugees have to face. Providing a safe, supportive space in which people can rediscover their abilities and regain their confidence to be active members of society.
- Giving priority to children, young people under 25 and their families, and those who have been in the UK for less than 10 years.
- Providing initial training for refugees working for the Centre in psychotherapy, counselling, administration or other skills useful in the organisation, to encourage re-entry into the job-market and society in general.

Over 21 years of its existence RTC offered psychoanalytic expertise and education in the delivery of an integrated and user-friendly mental health service for people who have endured considerable trauma and forced displacement. The Centre provided psychotherapy, counselling and associated treatments to refugees and asylum seekers were possible in people own language, if patient wish so. The Centre endeavours to help people to deal with and overcome psychological problems in a creative, supportive, respectful and containing environment in which they are better able to understand their feelings and experiences, and through this to feel more content about themselves. This provides people an opportunity to regain confidence, learn new skills and find the resilience they may have lost to enduring trauma and feeling empower to ease the process of immigrations and reintegration. In particular we are eager to help ease the demanding and intricate processes of transition many traumatised people have to face before they are able to become integrated, economically strong and productive members of the new society.

In addition to psychoanalytic psychotherapy and psychodynamic counselling, RTC also in the past have provided:

- Bi-lingual support outreach community development workers, who provide a more active style of support to people in coping with practical issues related to the processes of resettlement. The support workers also do outreach work to build links with refugee communities.
- A mentoring project that is one-to-one session work to support patients in the process of adapting to a new environment, to improve their English language as well as help children and young people to understand their school work.
- Training in intercultural psychoanalytical psychotherapy from foundation and introduction to master and clinical doctorate/PhD level.
- Provision of support and supervision for clinicians working within health services who needed specialist supervision.

Those worked at the RTC think that the following values lie at the heart of the organisation and its success. These values are an integral part of all its work:

- respect and recognition;
- development of staff and values contributions made;
- serving patient and the wider community;
- accountability;
- equality of opportunities for us; and
- fairness.

Each person at RTC incorporate these values into all aspects of work, as the expression of these values fundamentally transforms the establishment of both internal and external relationships as well as the organisation as a whole. Having said this, due to some changes in management, the restrictive process of Covid-19 and a lack of funding affecting the continuation of provision of services and training, but therapeutic interventions to aid refugees and asylum seekers at a smaller scale continued. Services like RTC in the UK and more so in London needed to continue. This is organisation with more than two decades of fostering and developing a therapeutic culture that restores connections with people who have endured persecution, imprisonment, torture and other forms of human right violations and displacement. Development and implementation of intercultural psychoanalytic approach at RTC is integrated the human rights into the therapeutic services for refugees and asylum seekers, by identifying a layer of resilience often may not be recognised during therapy, establishing therapeutic relationships that assume no imbalance of power to ensure fairness between patient and therapist by understanding and working with the socio-cultural circumstances of refugees and asylum seekers.

The RTC core service as specialist psychotherapy and associated treatments, based on an assessment of the needs of individuals and families that is based on the idea that:

- Services are inspired by feedback from the people we serve.
- Maintaining a dominant idea of childhood as a universalised and (paradoxically) very individualised construct that is built on notions of vulnerability and incompetence has led to interventions that, unintentionally, undermine children's resilience and denigrate their capacity.
- Focussing on children and adults' resilience, aspiration and capacity – rather than focussing on deficits- while working to reconstruct and restore a social identity and a sense of normality.
- The human rights are supported by our devotion to use negative experiences to create a positive outcome. In our view, if patients (both children and adults) are to be helped to overcome highly stressful experiences, their views and perspectives need to be treated with respect.
- To be the source of learning and strength, not a weakness, viewing peoples' potential resourcefulness is not to sanction their exposure to adversity, or to deny that some children, and indeed adults, may be rendered very vulnerable.

The RTC approach questions normative ideas about childhood weakness. We question whether a focus on children's vulnerabilities is the most effective way of supporting self-esteem and self-efficacy in adverse circumstances. In this sense:

- The service is not led by stereotypical notions of social norms, values, dynamics and power structures.

- The focus on the need to contextualise and foresee suitability of our services for people we set ourselves to serve and to give greater attention to ethnographic needs of people we are serving.
- To assure greater resiliency and sustainability and closer social and cultural adaptation for the community we serve.

At the RTC we are proud to have been able to fill some of these gaps over the past twenty years by providing much needed intercultural and bilingual services to refugees and asylum seekers who have endured trauma. During this period the work of the RTC has created an evidence base and framed the principles that have shaped the progress in the mental health of people we serve. I am proud to have witnessed the Centre's growth into something much more than the provision of therapy services. Through clinical interventions, research, policy analysis, community support workers community, group work, mentoring, parenting workshops and clinical training we witness powerful change to a path that resonates with best values. Having said this, there is still a long way to go before a mental health service for refugee and asylum seekers can meet the needs. The foundation of mental health for refugees and asylum seekers as well as other black and ethnic minorities, sexual minorities as well as people on low incomes, single parents and marginalised members of society can only starts through addressing the inequality and lack of fairness, asking for change and be part of the change.

The RTC policy development is focussed in areas associated with refugees and human rights, intercultural psychoanalytic psychotherapy, resilience and community engagement. We work with a range of regional, national and international networks in support of this activity and trust that communication between agencies and productive partnerships between refugee communities is essential to mobilising change. Examples of our networks are not limited to, but include, The Refugee Therapy Practitioners Forum, Psychologists working with Refugees and Asylum Seekers (PsyRAS), United Kingdom Council of Psychotherapy (UKCP) – Council for Psychoanalysis and Jungian Analysis (CPJA), European Alliance, the World Association of Cultural Psychiatry (WACP) and the International Rehabilitation Council for Torture Victims (IRCT). We have taken an active role in policy debates through these networks by being part of committees, attending conferences and symposia. The Centre worked to influence central government in particular the Home Office, engaging in research project and being corporate members of the National Asylum Stakeholder Forum where items associated with improving the immigration and asylum system are discussed.

The support workers project

The core activity at the Centre is to provide psychological support, based on monitoring and evaluations a significant proportion of people do have practical issues that need to be addressed. The community development support workers were a response to these needs. Employment for example usually is not addressed with refugee and asylum seekers patients, and therefore support for employability is limited dealing with surface symptoms as opposed to deep rooted issues such as those associated with post-traumatic stress.

Campaigning

The Centre campaigning work is focussed on supporting those who face human rights violations and persecution, by engaging with the UK government, local MPs and journalists to highlight the need for change. Another way of influencing involving, speaking and presenting at events and symposia to highlight the need for alternative approaches to working therapeutically, providing data that psychoanalytic interventions with refugees and asylum seekers is much better suited. We advocate for change of clinical and theoretical development items associated with intercultural psychoanalytic psychotherapeutic interventions alongside working to identify resilience as a factor in working with the trauma associated with torture and other forms of human rights violations. We also are contributing to the field by writing articles in Journals and media debates that are presented in psychoanalytic and psychotherapeutic publications as a means of promoting the need for cultural sensitive interventions that support individuals' basic human rights, including refugee.

Research

RTC research work draws on clinical expertise and excellence and is led, as with other aspects of our work, through evaluation and outcome of patients. We may for instance during the therapeutic process identify the need to develop new ways for client intervention or gaps in knowledge that would benefit not only those particular person but agencies working in areas affected by human rights. We were running research on trauma, torture and dissociation as an ongoing clinical research into the effects of trauma and types of dissociations. The main research question was: 'Why is it that some people respond to trauma with a successful act of dissociation, leaving the organisation of their world reasonably intact, while others experience fragmentation of the self and of their perception of the world?' The methodology chosen was observing cases to identify causal factors associated with the pragmatic phenomenon in a flexible, but rigorous manner systematically, documenting any changes and the pattern of change made in patients (i.e. the change that comes immediately after an interpretation or in the form of a dream in the following sessions).

Evaluating the data we have identified four key factors as important:

- sense of self;
- psychic space;
- a listening other; and
- dissociation.

In the clinical interventions all psychoanalytic psychotherapists continuously examine presenting issues and the changes to identify how and what are the connections between these four and how to identify what make the person resilient. For example, the notion of a good enough therapist that I term a 'listening other' is connected with having a 'psychic space' and with psychic space comes a 'sense of self'. The work on fostering resilience shown to be informed by promoting self-esteems and opening up positive opportunities and by using innate self-righting mechanism to transform and make change, focusing on reducing the personal impact of risk experiences and negative chain reactions, opening up positive cognitive processing of negative experiences, to build an ability to form relationships with social competence and to develop a sense of self and autonomy, that will build psychic space to plan and hope with a sense of purpose and future. The trauma experienced becomes a memory of the past.

Monitoring and evaluation

Measuring the progress by monitoring the delivery and the outcomes in the process was through regular data collection that is gathered from patients' sessions as well as refugee steering committees (two steering group, a group of leaders of refugee communities and the clinical steering group), the focus groups consists of therapists agreed to participate in the research actively, assessments, every ten sessions progress reports, closing summary and feedback. Patients also are asked to give feedback on their experience of the quality of services provided and whether the service received is appropriate to their needs and for suggestions and comments for service improvement. For the purpose of this research we gather information such as the number of patients referred and assessed the number of sessions and frequency provided, the patterns of individual attendance via attendance logs. In addition a written closing summary from therapists to ensure the treatment has been effectively followed through, which is kept in a main file. Results of this process are analysed in a strictly confidential manner by me as the clinical lead. The results are shared and discussed with the managers and staff members concerned – information such as lessons learned about what has been successful and what are the challenges to overcome and where possible the planning and implementation process is modified according to the outcome. In terms of the monitoring and evaluation associated with change in patients the following was identified:

- Increased confidence and self-esteem.
- Improved concentration and attention, improved memory.
- Making of new friends and integration.
- Reduction in anxiety and depression.
- Increase in positive hopes and aspirations for the future.
- Increased ability to use English in daily life.
- Learning how to access statutory and voluntary services without fears.
- Engagement with education, training and employment, paid and voluntary.
- Reduction in feelings of isolation, marginalisation, anger and frustrations due to feeling of perceived prejudice and racism.
- Improvement in relationships.

These were evidence of the effects of the therapeutic intervention through patients improvement, with the majority reporting significant reductions of negative thoughts and feelings, and therapists progress reports on reductions in clinical symptoms of depression, anxiety, post traumatic stressors and other psychosocial stresses such as social exclusion, unemployment, homelessness, immigration matters, lack of English language, sense of isolations and loneliness, feeling unwanted and rejected and cultural alienations that were preventing people to work and settle in their new environment. In addition, therapists collect in-house designed comprehensive assessment forms, including PHQ9 and GAD7. The PHQ9 helps to facilitate the recognition of common mental health stresses patients were presenting, including depression. Its regular review over time was helpful to monitor changes in patients. GAD-7 is helpful to identify anxiety, panic, social anxiety and post-traumatic stress symptoms.

For over 21 years the Refugee Therapy Centre has been the source for the provision of intercultural therapeutic interventions in London and beyond. Led by the renowned expert in the field, RTC offers refugees, asylum seekers and destitutes space to think and to find possible solution for psychological stressors they are under due to the past experiences, indeed the anxiety and uncertainty about the immigration and other matters in the new environment. The resilience focus approaches employed at the RTC clinical intervention focuses on positive, not deficit, allowing people to gain or regain resiliency and feel in control of the new life and providing and learn tools to manage life in the new environment. The group work we developed provided various ways and levels for psychological recovery for those experiencing anxiety and stress-related difficulties and involves the active participation of patients (and their parents, in the case of children) in the process of recovery; breaking the ring of isolation was the first steps to recovery. The intercultural psychoanalytical therapeutic intervention resilience base approach utilises to help modify thought patterns, carefully expose patients to situations which have been creating fear and enables people to experience success moving on in life. The intercultural practice gives us the flexibility to focus the intervention where patients need it most. For instance, we know anxiety diminishes the person's ability to participate in typical daily activities. At the RTC therapists will conduct sessions in way patients feel at ease to look at the cause of the anxiety. By systematically and carefully helping patients to talk about the painful or fearful situations the Centre aims to reduce the discomfort and symptoms patients feel.

Chapter 2

Assessment or initial interview

The ability to create a safe environment and to get an idea of the patient's frame of reference is a major clinical skill. When working with refugees, in the initial assessment the analyst needs to cover the full social, political and psychological disturbance, which may last for more than one meeting. Sullivan (1946, 1953) writes about the psychiatric interview, and its purpose as elucidating characteristic patterns of living of the subject. Sullivan (1946) believes that, if consideration is given to the nonverbal but nonetheless primarily vocal aspects of the exchange, it is actually feasible to make a crude formulation of many people within an hour and a half. In such assessment, the analyst needs to take care not to imply rigidity, but to retain flexibility towards the varying concerns and communication patterns of different individuals. The paramount objective is to establish rapport with the patient in a working alliance.

From the first encounter with a patient, as analyst we usually begin to form a working image of the person. This working image will not necessarily be divulged to the patient, but is a set of hypotheses concerning the patient's strengths, coping strategies and limitations. Thus working with refugees, the poverty of their ability to convey what is going on in their mind and their life in the past as well as in the present must be appreciated, before making a diagnosis or further treatment. We need to be very sensitive to a refugee patient's identity and personality, because at time a refugee patient may be incapable of verbalising her or his experiences. It is challenging to hypothesise and to form an opinion of whether a refugee's mental disturbance arises out of traumatic experiences or is a specific clinical characteristic. In other words, is it the result of external or internal reality or both and to what level. We need also to determine whether disturbances arise from development or from a cultural belief system. Coltart (1988) says, the assessment interview may be the most momentous occasion in the patient's life. The experience of paying attention as a good listening other may be quite unique for a patient, and can be a deeply positive and be the start a therapeutic dyad on this basis that is if we do not make an early interpretation. The interpretation for bringing attention to those aspects of the patient of which the patient is unaware or wishes to continue being unaware is not helpful.

DOI: 10.4324/9781003401322-3

Hinshelwood (1991) indicated that clinical material is best approached as pictures in three areas of object relationships: first, the current life situation; second, infantile object relations, as described in the patient's history, or hypothesised from what is known; and third, the relationship with the assessor which, to all intents and purposes, is the beginning of a transference. Working interculturally, I would summarise the central themes of the patient's current and past life situation, and their perception of internal and external effects, in the initial interview, as well as the patient's resiliencies and vulnerabilities, and assign a developmental level to the patient's personality organisation. By the end of the assessments, I like to have covered the main features of the patient's current circumstances, family background, detailed developmental history, especially psychosexual history, history of major losses and trauma, dreams, main areas of interest and aptitude; and to have some idea about sources of both stress and support. Where relevant, I also gather some knowledge of past psychiatric history, including history of hospital admission, psychotropic drugs, suicide attempts and substance use, as well as mental states, such as depressive, obsessional and psychotic phenomena.

Try to recognise the distinction between Oedipal (three person neurotic difficulties, and object-related) or pre-Oedipal (two person borderline and narcissistic problems, as fundamental in early development), as well as looking for strengths of ego, self or drive. It is also basic for my practice to assess gender and its implication in the initial encounter, specifically when working with refugees. We need also to look at gender and power, and maternal and paternal relationships in the specific cultural context of the individual and group. It is my view that in order to analyse the mechanisms which control all aspects of gender differences, we need to outline the concept of femininity and masculinity. Generally speaking, some characteristics are gender-specific in all cultures: women and men have different experiences, relationship and concerns. As analyst we need and must understand and work with these differences. Consider the interaction between the intra-psychic and the social reality of one's life; the ability to differentiate the internal world from external reality in a refugee in therapy. Some issues we usually take for granted may play a major part in making clear what particular issue may effect patients, for instance what gender means in a particular culture; how it operates; and how it is negotiated in personal relationships in the specific culture; what effect it has on patients' conscious and unconscious; as well as the level of integration and its effect on the process of resettlement in the new environment. For example in all cultures, sexual and physical abuse is associated with great humiliation and fear of permanent damage. But, the psychological consequences of sexual violence depend on the culture or subculture, their social role and religion. In some cultures, deflowering may result in the women no longer being acceptable as a marriage candidate. In other cultures, rape may result in a woman becoming stigmatised and ostracised in community, and even by her own family. What would be the result of sexual abuse and rape in one's daily life therefore cannot be simplified, and we need to take a broad and diverse view based on patients' presentation. In my clinical works I learned that there are distinctions between rape by prison officials as part of torture, and in other circumstances such as known person or stranger within community. The person abused by rape often presents complaints such as nervousness, insomnia, depression, reduced self-esteem and feelings of humiliation; but where sexual abuse was part of torture, further mental problems can interfere with cognitive function, such as lack of concentration, memory disturbances, flashbacks, nightmares, intrusive thought, lack of trust, suspicion and delusions as well as sexual dysfunction.

Looking at gender differences in all societies, both nature and culture influence the definition of any individual. There is a distinction between the consequences of sexual violence in Western and non-western culture and society, especially for women. Culture determines how the individual, as a man or a woman, thinks, acts, perceives and feels. For example in some cultures, having a boy is honourable, but having a girl is shameful, and the man's role is to protect family honour. Generally looking at a fundamentalist religious community, women expected to be strong, and to be kept under control to prevent them from tempting the men to forsake their social and religious duties. In such a cultural perspective, rape is blamed on the woman, and can result in social rejection; as a result women who are raped by and large decide to keep silent as a protective shell. In particular, in some Middle Eastern, Asian and some other Muslim families, women are expected to be dependent on men (fathers and brothers before marriage, and husbands after marriage); and men are expected to control women and children. In these cultures, the only way to enter adulthood for women is marriage. Also in such cultures, behaviour such as homosexuality or freedom to choose the partner openly is out of the question. Women having sex before marriage are considered abnormal, and will not be tolerated. Women must exert self-control even in their private life, for the sake of family honour. Family, especially men's honour not to damaged and be replaced by shame if a female member of the family is raped. In such cultures, a raped women is not seen as a victim of abuse and violation, but simply a 'dirty women', a 'whore'; so the raped woman learns not to tell their male members of family as their 'protector', what has happened to them. This experience remains a secret shared only with the rapist, in the hope that she will forget it; believing that knowledge of her rape will kill her, or destroy her family. Therefore she carries the burden alone, in order to survive and protect the family. Such woman in isolated mind may build an internal relationship with perpetuator that of course will have a destructive potential.

I will not go into much detail about cultural differences here as in this book my focus is upon a group of refugee patients who have endured external trauma in adult life as a result of socio-political environment as well as whose biological needs for nurture and comfort were not adequately met. Also, for many the mothers or primary carers never related to them beyond simple caretaking. They never smiled at their children, had no pleasure from playing with them or in their emerging sense of aliveness. We can hypothesise that the mothers used their children as transitional objects. In turn, the children's emotional development became fixated in the in-between transition space. This fixation led to specific types of character structure that can leads to ego defects. So, in many people I worked in groups the early development did not form a smooth continuum that acquired adaptive ego states. So, there is extensive gap in layers of the psychic apparatus which manifested themselves as defective modulating elements. Patients show behaviour marked divergences of being sane, sensitive and rational, indeed, at time exhibited a peculiar kind of fragmentation or splitting. There are many patients initial presentations of problems in the group can be paradoxical which can lead to a treatment impasse caused by an imbrication's of psychopathology and various characteristics attribution. From psychoanalytic theory and perspectives it is not difficult to compare the mother's attitude toward her infant child has some similarity to the low-keyed objective analytic neutrality. But, in my view in the start of working with such patients we require different modes of relating which indicate that the analyst is, unlike the mother, listen carefully and concerned with their patient's developing autonomy for the external world. These variations in treatment are not modifications or deviations from psychoanalysis; they are rather elements of the analytic process necessary for the treatment of specific types of psychopathology. Just as each patient is unique and the transference manifests itself in a particular way and we as the analyst can think and decide certain interpretations, the variations of technique address the construction of a containing and holding environment appropriate in working with traumatised refugee patients within the group not to encourage unnecessary conflicts.

My way of intercultural psychoanalytic assessment and diagnoses based on patient presentations are focus on:

1   Early childhood narrative and individual character formations.
2   Trauma exposure in early and adult life and level of resiliency or vulnerability that is perceived self-control and quality of life, and severity of traumatic event/s.
3   Depressive and anxiety symptoms by individual's presentation without pre-assumption, indeed without the need of fitting with particular structured assessment tools.

My approach for assessing participants for a group focuses on developing and overseeing an individualised evaluation of patient to be invited to group I also focus on:

a   transference here-and-now coping skills;
b   community reintegration; and
c   therapeutic exposure and narrative reconstruction of unresolved trauma potentially can be from early developmental process.

In many of cases I worked with in the group the prevalence of early child-hood trauma in vulnerable patients was quite high. Early trauma and later history and vulnerabilities were shown to be close to 100% interrelated. Involving variables that I will try to address by presenting in brief vignettes both in individual assessment process and in the group and to describe a distribution that involves a number of random but related variables analyses of variance for repeated symptom presentation of dissociative types which provides evidence to measure each individual classification and history of early childhood trauma as between patients independent variables, and time of presentations (i.e. in assessment process or early intervention versus post one year intervention in the group) with each patients independent unpredictability or adaptability within the group interactions.

I can think about the idea of Winnicott (1958) that at the preliminary stages of the development of mother–infant interaction, anxiety and the dread of annihilation are also closely connected to the notion of holding. It is holding that enables the baby to become a self. Winnicott (1958) refers to this as the 'continuity of being', the alternative to being is reacting, and reacting interrupts being and annihilates. Further, Winnicott viewed the root of the tiny baby's terror in terms of being able just 'to be'. His idea differs from Kleinian theory, as he considered that aggression and destructiveness were not a function or projection of the death instinct, as the new-born baby could not hate until it was able to comprehend the notion of wholeness. Within this context the capacity of hate for a child, can occur after the initial holding stage. According to Winnicott in this phase the ego changes over from an unintegrated state to a structured integration, and so the child becomes able to experience anxiety associated with disintegration. He con-siders a healthy development at this stage the infant retains the capacity for re-experiencing these unintegrated states depends on the continuation and endurance of reliable maternal care. The main function of Winnicott holding environment therefore is the reduction of impingements to which the infant must react with consequential annihilation of personal being.

Assessing single traumatic event and repeated or ongoing trauma

There is a distinction between single and repeated traumas. Single shocking events such as earthquakes, hurricanes, floods, volcanoes, plane crashes, robbery, rape and homicide can produce shock and trauma reactions. But the traumatic experiences that result in the most serious mental health problems are usually prolonged and repeated, and at times can continued over years of a person's life. The single unexpected direct trauma may cause typical symptoms of relentless flashbacks, persistent avoidance and increased arousal. It does not appear to strain the massive denials, psychic numbing, self-anaesthesia or a personality problems characterised in so called PTSD symptoms and diagnosis, though it can impair some areas of psychological functioning.

The complex traumas, which are continuous and repetitive ordeals that gain prolonged and appalling anticipation in one area of human functioning, produce the most severe effects on mental health. Such experience may create enormous defence mechanisms of repression, denial, dissociation, somatisation, self-anaesthesia, depersonalisation, self-hypnosis, identification with the aggressor and aggression against the self. The impairment in emotional processing includes a sense of constant anger and frustration, and deep sadness and fear, which is all quite common in refugees' experience. Toleration of prolonged stressors, inflicted on a person with intention to abuse such as torture is much more complex than the toleration of accidents or natural disasters. If harm was inflicted deliberately in the context of a social correlation, such as torture, the predicament is greater than that of an accident. In situations where the injury is caused deliberately in a relationship by a person whom the injured party become helpless and tortured, or by ongoing abuse by a parent or caregiver in relation to the child, the effect of trauma can be horrendous and unspeakable. Sadistic abuses on the subject of interpersonal violence by person/s as an eruption of passions in the severest forms are those inflicted deliberately. Premeditated cruelty such as torture can be more atrocious and terrifying for long term and more injurious.

Cross-generational transmission

Transmitted trauma are different between persons or generations with different mechanisms, such as symbiosis, empathy, attachment, enmeshment, personal or collective identification, projective identification, introjections, dependency, co-dependency, interdependency, parenting, compensation and acculturation. Individual coexists in a system or a network of intertwine relationships that transmit the effects of different significant events. An example is shared psychotic disorder; development of a delusion in a person in the context of a close relationship with another person(s) who has an already established delusion (DSM IV, 297.3; American Psychiatric Association, 1994). Traumas can have similar effects on persons in relationships, or within strong collective identity, even if they did not suffer the trauma themselves. In this context, trauma can happen not only to one person, but also to a social unit, to a community, or sometimes to a whole society (e.g. genocide, civil war, ethnic cleansing). However, the transmission of trauma does not automatically always occur; for the same reason as an extreme traumatic event may not necessarily result in post-trauma symptoms in a resilient person. The transmission can happen from one person to another or to a connected group that has been affected by trauma and collectively lost their healthy defences and coping mechanisms. There are also indirect traumas and its effects which may transmit within a family system across generations, such as domestic or other type of violence, physical abuse and incest in some families. The intergenerational continuity of those family patterns is often expressed by young children becoming violent and perpetrators, or colluding with the victim's role, repeating the intergenerational cycle of victim and perpetrator of violence.

From psychoanalytic perspectives, projective identification is helpful in identifying the history of trauma inflicted and possible mechanism that can facilitate the transmission of unresolved traumatic experiences. Projective identification in the context of parent-child relationships involves the parent's recruitment of the child to perform a particular role for the parent's externalised unconscious fantasies, and is thought to harm a child by weakening the child's capacity to experience his or her own subjective awareness, insight and feelings as an acceptable reality. A child in the parent's projective fantasies lead to a collapse of the potential space within the parent–child relationship that allow for the development of child's autonomy, though this transmission is not automatic.

Collective cross-generational trauma transmission across generations can be divided into collective traumas which is more a collective complex trauma as it is inflicted on a group of people that have specific group identity or affiliation to collective culture such as ethnicity, colour, national origin, religion and political beliefs. Historical information prior to traumatisation and the intensity of traumatic exposure including the effects is important. Historical trauma can predispose the individual to poorly respond to later traumas. Prior traumatisation is generally associated with more symptoms and longer recovery. There is also the multigenerational transmission of political or structural violence that constitutes extreme social disparities created by generating deprived social structures.

Chronic and ongoing threats to secure life many asylum seekers are experiencing can either stimulate or overwhelm their sense of survival. This can disturb their values and processing from one to all areas of psychological functioning. Furthermore, the effects of deprivation by poverty, rights, citizenship and immigration status may cause further trauma and lead to demoralisation, socioeconomic disadvantage, lower levels of achievement and an increased level of socio-psychological problems. Poverty may also convert into the halting of intellectual development and into educational deprivation for many refugee and asylum seekers, especially children and young people, even for those who have no apparent biological restrictions to learning. The direct and indirect cross-generational consequences of such structural violation of basic human right can be devastating and enduring to any human being. This type of ongoing traumatic condition is the type which can and, in many cases will, transmit across generations.

A few brief vignettes of patients during the assessments for group

A woman I shall call Anna, a senior social worker, referred herself for support as she felt she cannot cope with her work and family demands. In the first meeting she said that she grew up with very caring parents in a stable working-class neighbourhood in an inner-city area in her country of origin. She had satisfactory relationships with her siblings and was strongly indicating that her childhood was wonderful, but in her adult life, and especially since she started to work in London, she can't understand why she constantly feel hurt in relationships with others, and why she constantly feels that she has to take care of others, causing more work and creating inconvenience. She gives example of colleagues who repeatedly arrived to their shift sometimes up to two hours late, with excuses of traffic or childcare, and she always with a smile says 'OK, no worries', while she is boiling of anger inside with long shift as a duty social worker who cannot stop until handover to the next shift colleague. I asked of her childhood. She said that her father was the breadwinner working long hours in a factory and her mother due to an accident at work become disabled, and Anna and some of her siblings had to become carers from a very young age. She recalls learning to cook tomato from age of six. I made a gentle interpretation that until now she really cannot understand her childhood with her mother serious disability and absent father was not as wonderful as she thinks it was, only because her parents were not abusive to her and her siblings physically. She without being defensive understood how much of her past within this context was alive in the present and how much of her caring nature to disable mother affected her in relating to others in the caring professions. She cannot leave duty shift unattended and at risk because her colleagues are late. She was pleased to have insight of her behaviour and realised she can set a clearer boundary with her colleagues without feeling that she is neglecting clients or her colleague. I was impressed by her and thought Anna is a suitable candidate for the group. I proposed to her and she accepted to join, but hesitantly. She asked if I could see her individually. I said I think it will be more beneficial for her to be in group. She accepted.

   Another patient, Betty, an anxious and nervous nurse with composed way of talking with no emotion and persistent quantifiable dimension of her personal and professional life experience, was concerned that she is 39 years old and she had not yet accomplished any of her main goals in life. Betty also presented her childhood as good and described her problem was started when she reached seventeen in her last year of her schooling and before going to university. She with prominence stress revealed that in her childhood and in her country did not suffer as much, because at least she did not have the challenges of different language and different culture. She was talking non-stop with the intention of convincing me that her account of herself is absolutely right and she wanted a quick fix from me for her ongoing anxieties; she said she is very keen to see me but did not want the psychoanalytic silliness. At this point, I decided to give a brief interpretation. I asked her if she sees language as separate from other aspects of her or other cultures. She immediately with politeness cut me off and said, you are absolutely right, language is an element of culture, but what I was trying to tell you was that cultures and languages are not unrelated to my anxiety and nervousness. I stopped her and suggested there might be other matters or experiences that she has endured that at the moment she preferred not to address them to protect herself from further anxiety and possible total breakdown. She burst into tears and nodded positively. I gently responded, saying that is OK, this shows her strength and knowledge of her own ability and awareness of her vulnerability and limitation which is good and positive. I said she can talk about other concerning matters as and when she is ready. She looked at me with content and a painful smile and tears was dropping from her eyes. She said thank you for listening to me and understanding me. I didn't think she will be candidate for group immediately with that level of anxiety. I told her this meeting was to consider her joining a group I am setting up and I do like to invite her to join the group I am setting up but not with this level of stress that she currently has. We arranged to meet again in couple of months, and I said I will refer her to one of my colleague to be seen individually first. She initially was resistant but with further explorations, she agreed to go to eight sessions I proposed after that together we decide if it is best for her to continue remaining in the individual therapy further or she join group the group. She agreed on this.

My intentions for presenting these two vignettes of assessments are to demonstrate that with careful attention, right questions on the right time, and gentle interpretations and if needed confrontation of contradictions in presenting problem we can facilitate an environment for patients to thoughtfully and vigilantly address the emotional struggles of fears, anger, hatred and confusion they might be feeling or facing to be addressed and guardedly gain insight about situations. As the analyst, I learned that I must avoid the temptation to try to impose my version of normality or abnormality to the patient. For instance, if I think forgiveness and letting go is a healthy approach, I should not intimidate patients with my view or present my view as the correct or normal one, especially when patient idealising me as good object in transference. My job as analyst is to help the patient overcome defensiveness and find answers. I see our job as analysts to strive to help patients to overcome their traumatic experience by use of us as the object, and to assess the patterns of patient attachment, the defensiveness, strengths and weakness with transference and very gentle interpretations.

I learned from Ezriel (1950) who undertook assumed scientific testing of psychoanalytic theory and practice in his analytic group work. His group setting approach tended to be as if he was working with one patient, seeking unifying themes, assumptions, and trends in the interaction of the members. He restricts his activity as an analyst to two basic tenets:

1   Everything the patients say or do is related to the analyst.
2   The only intervention of the group analyst is to interpret, and with each interpretation to focus on and reinforce the view that all intrapsychic and interpersonal behaviour of all the patients is always analyst-oriented, always transferential. He later (Ezriel, 1956) explained that in his group work he 'refrained from making a reference to the past and used solely here and now interpretations' (p. 48). He emphasised that a strict here and now approach will allow the experimental study of the behaviour of an individual in the psychoanalytic intervention. He concludes that 'a here and now approach without reference to the patient's past, over-comes objections which are commonly brought against the possibility of using the psycho-analytic session as an experimental situation in which hypotheses about human behaviour can be tested' (p. 48).

The vignettes I presented in this chapter for the process of assessment are intended to provide an understanding of complex issues and encompassing to particular types of traumata and what is already known to patient con-scious level. I tried to provide contextual analysis of a limited number of events or conditions and relations between them. I used qualitative method to provide the basis for the application of ideas and extension of techniques, as an analytic practice and inquiry for exploration. Vignettes I consider as methods of enquiry and as data I applied to establish a firm focus to which I will be used and referred to throughout the work with all patients and in each group participants. It was of course clear each patient presented com-plex and difficult life events, wanting to understand or resolve traumas that they had endured in the way they understood prior to seeking help. Each patient's presentation brought many interrelated elements and factors con-nected to their political, social, historical, and personal issues. These provide a range of possibilities for questions on each case presented as contributing factors in the group, while each also remaining as an individual and single case with specific life events. A key strength of the method I used here involves using multiple clinical data in brief vignettes in the process of assessments and techniques I used to identify participants for each specific groups. In the process, represents a contribution toward the systematic and empirical investigation of psychoanalytic assessments and treatments in the group. I used object relations theory within intercultural approach that allows the translation of clinical data into amenable qualitative form and empirical means to test theoretically and clinically within intercultural psychoanalytic process in working with people who have endured external trauma. Outcome of groups for me insinuate that subjecting the traditional psychoanalytic case illustration to systematic and regular inquiry can establish empirical scientific methods for intercultural psychoanalytic group intervention.

The psychoanalysis assessments on individuals for forming an analytic group and focusing on individual potential group participants provided here by vignettes is important for forming a group ongoing review of patient characteristics and the problematic aspects of life events at the point of entry, patterns of attachments and relating to me as the analysts and others outside the consulting room. are equally important for group work Deconstructing the psychopathology of a patient in the process of assessments, using a variety of methodological efforts to uncover the roots the presenting symptoms, while ratifying and validating psychoanalysis and empiricism in general, eases the process of integrating into the groups for all participants. The relationship between the presenting problems by each and collective patients and my intervention with gentle interpretations within the groups are main evidence that I used as my clinical data, made careful notes, classified, and cross-referenced and delaminated over the course of the writing about group work. The raw data also used for interpretations in order to find linkages between the explore and examine objective and the therapeutic outcomes. The case study method, with its use of multiple data collection and psychoanalytic techniques, that I have used systematically in my work and with vignettes for this book, provides strengths to clinical outcome. The analysis of the data necessitated a move beyond the initial question, but provided accurate and reliable findings. Throughout the evaluation and analysis of outcome, room was left for new learning and insights and further research questions. The narratives of assessments presented on all patients for group participations are objectively based on collection of clinical data and is not based on my intuition as the analyst. The method I used involves looking at clinical material as empirical data rather than an illustration of my preferred theory. With this method the findings from the group interventions provide one kind of validation for psychoanalytic reconstructions, making it possible to provide a satisfactory degree of certainty in the attempt to integrate the patient's psychic truth with historical truth that Freud (1937) refers to. The use of reconstruction is an important dimension of the psychoanalytic technique that helps me greatly to gain understanding of how an adult or part of an adult has remained a disturbed child with that particular psychopathology. The significance of reconstruction is important for restoring personality, continuity and cohesion, and for explaining neurotic repetition as it has developed in life and in the analytic transference. Freud (1905, 1917, 1937) himself sought validity of his discoveries by emphasising the importance of establishing an agreement between analytic reconstructions and the results of naturalistic child observation. Ahumada (1994, 1997) in contrast explains his view on the inductive workings of clinical psychoanalysis, in which mainly pragmatic facts evolve within a pragmatic relational field in ways which allow cognitions to emerge. He emphasised that his use of the term 'induction' is meant in the wider sense in which Whewell (1858), Quine (1961), Russell (1948) and Von Wright (1957) conceive it, and not in the restrictive sense that Braithwaite (1953) or Grünbaum (1984) have used it. Ahumada says that the distinction between facts and theories is only relative. He cited Von Wright (1960), who, contrary to inductive generalisation, operates on the saying that the future will differ from the past. If the evolution of psychic facts in psychoanalysis brings unconscious processes to the preconscious-conscious domain of the no counter induction becomes central to the psychoanalytic method as far as the patient is concerned. He assumes that what the therapist will describe interpretively as psychic facts are mainly the ways the patient puts into the unconscious patterns of the patient reaches an apparent insight into clinical facts when, helped along by the descriptive drawing transferred by the interpretations attains an important and powerful position by double or multiple observations in individual concrete instances of the falsification of an unconscious.

The same objectives later led Lichtenberg & Lieberman (1983) and Stern (1985) to produce evaluations of infant research findings on analytic developmental propositions. This utilisation of reconstruction surely will be helpful to identify the linkage between historical events and the patient's intrapsychic structure – through the process of interpretation and response to the here and now in transference, as well as the linkage between past and present, childhood and adult psychopathology. Reconstruction may not always follow from the transference; it is rather an inferential and integrative act from resistance and amnesia, which may also be the result of substance by chemical processes of memories, and biological syntheses interpretations for missing memory and gaps in history – specifically trauma related history. The reconstructive integration identifies patterns and the interrelationship aspects of patients' personality and the intrapsychic configurations consequences, rather than isolated conflicts and experiences. Therefore, developmental influences are more important than actual historical facts that contribute to the formation, testing, and validation of psychoanalytic treatments and theory.

Findings on the therapeutic efficacy of the interpretation and reconstruction of repressed past unconscious conflicts and trauma have been observed by being an ongoing analytical 'listening other' (Alayarian 2015). I give attention to the conflictual process that Greenacre (1956, 1960) talked about:

> Specific 'fantasies' which persist until adult life are rarely only 'typical' fantasies, common to all infantile development, but rather those typical ones which have been given special strength, form and pressure for repetition through having been confirmed by external events.
>
> (Greenacre, 1956, p. 643)

This was helpful to contains all the components of conflict and shaped both the patient's and my conflict as the analyst in every moment. The mutual responsiveness that develops between patient and I, which stems from a complex conflictual object relationship, is similar to any other object relationship, in which transference and countertransference at all times simultaneously facilitate and interfere with the analytic work. I find presenting vignette to be useful to illustrate these related phenomena, including the use of signal conflict, the benign, and vulnerable or, at times, negative transference and countertransference; the function of my countertransference and patient use of repetition compulsion and projection at time in response to my interpretations. By doing so, one's affects, thoughts, and actions trace the shifting nature of the transference-resistance that help the level of the object relationship continuously being created between patient and I in our therapeutic dyad. In his book *Restoration of the Self*, Kohut (1977) expressed that in all he had written on the psychology of the self, he had purposely not defined the self. He knew that some would be critical of him for that omission. He explained that it had become impossible to base his work on his predecessors because he would have been entangled in a 'thicket' of similar, overlapping or identical terms and concepts, which did not carry the same meaning and were not employed as a part of the same conceptual context. He refers to a patient whose personality disturbance was marked by a vertical split in his personality. One fragment in this patient was characterised by a sense of superiority and messianic identification that resulted from a merger with his mother, who had idealised him and encouraged the grandiosity. He also refers to cognitive impenetrability and says 'introspectively or empathically perceived psychological manifestations are open to us' (ibid., p. 311). The self for Kohut is 'the way a person experiences himself as himself' (ibid., p. xv), a permanent mental structure consisting of feelings, memories, and behaviours that are subjectively experienced as being continuous in time and as being 'me'. The self is also a 'felt centre of independent initiative', and an 'independent recipient of impression', the centre of the individual's psychological universe (ibid., p. xv), and not simply a representation. He says 'our transient individuality also possesses a significance that extends beyond the borders of our life' (ibid., p. 180) and describes 'cosmic narcissism' which transcends the boundaries of the individual.

Along the same lines, Steiner (1993) discusses that neurotic, perverse, borderline and psychotic patients all have narcissistic structures in their personality. He termed this '*psychic retreat*' that is found with stuck patients, using the retreat in a transient and discretionary way:

> Patients who withdraw excessively to psychic retreats present major problems of technique. The frustration of having a stuck patient, who is at the same time out of reach, challenges the analyst, who has to avoid being driven either to give up in despair or to over-react and try to

overcome opposition ... retreat is achieved at the cost of isolation, stagnation and withdrawal, and some patients find such a state distressing
and complain about it. Others, however, accept the situation with resig-
nation, relief and at times defiance or triumph, so that it is the analyst
who has to carry the despair.

(Steiner, 1993, p. 131)

Steiner further suggests:

retreat is experienced as a cruel place and the deadly nature of the
situation is recognised by the patient, but more often the retreat is
idealised and represented as a pleasant and even ideal haven. Whether
idealised or persecutory, it is clung to as preferable to even worse
states.

(Steiner, 1993, p. 2)

He also talks about technical problems relating to the nature of interpretations and how they are likely to be received by the intensely frightened and
hostile patient who fears the abrupt and permanent loss of the 'psychic
retreat'. He offers some ideas to analysts in their attempts to stay with the
patient, and to understand more clearly 'what the stakes are' at critically
difficult points in the work. His discussion assists us in recognising and
understanding what is going on, and in being more open to those moments
in which we sometimes become drawn into supporting the patient's pathological organisation. He discusses how and when to interpret the transference
relationship to patients and to recognise when they are ready to receive them,
and how we need to judge this from careful observation of the patient's presentations. He explores the idea of the patient's capacity to understand what
it is they are doing, whether or not the projection first has to be taken up in
the analyst rather than from the patient. Once the perceived nature of the
object is explored, the conditions for deeper understanding can become possible. These differences in emphasis deeply influence how we intervene, and
whether or not our patient sees us as the analyst, as someone who can provide understanding. Steiner also outlines the delicate use of the countertransference, which he calls 'analyst-centred interpretations', with patients, as
a method of understanding, explain and clarify the patient's use of projective
identification. This, he suggests, enables the patient to explore his disturbed
perceptions of reality outside himself, located in analyst, and avoids the
problem of the patient's withdrawal and retreat when confronted by 'patient-
centred interpretations' that forcibly return projections to patients which may
be threatening and be perceived attacking with too much awareness too
quickly. He indicated that the patient often has a profound feeling of not
having an understanding object, and that is one reason for them to organise
a 'psychic retreat' in response to a world lacking in objects.

Tuckett (1994) argues that validation in the clinical process depends on being as clear about the hypotheses and suggests that in sessions, interpretation is mainly based on intuitive and 'quite spontaneous links arising from background orientations' (ibid., p. 1159). Tuckett rightly places emphasis on the importance of the patient's and analyst's external reality outside the session, a wider and more developed set of grounded hypotheses can be developed, intended to illuminate what seem to be the core issues that arise over time, and the core problems suffered by the patient.

Hinshelwood (1994), in a discussion about random control trials, suggests objectification in psychiatry is problematic. He indicates that the key requirement is an objective indicator of change in pathological signs such as blood levels of specific substances, bodily lumps etc. The primary focus in such practice is to objectively assess treatments on the basis of their impact on the same specific indicator, aiming to compare like with like. Crucial to this is the objective quantification of the independent and dependent variables with regard to patients' presentations that is central to psychoanalytic practice. In the psychoanalytic methods there are two ways in which patients produced their memories of the past: one was by recollecting in words; the other was by repeating, in some form, actual past events or phantasies. Repetition or re-creating in the relationship in the transference as an expressive act revealing contents of the patient's unconscious can become a cornerstone of psychoanalytic technique:

> It could be argued that this is perhaps the most important development in the clinical practice of psychoanalysis and more important than any of the multitude of developments in psychoanalytic theory, because the transference is the tool by which all the evidence and testing of the theory take place.
>
> (Hinshelwood, 1999, p. 13)

He further argues:

> The psychiatric drive to objectify symptoms and diagnoses takes place inevitably in a framework made up of social attitudes held by doctors, patients and society at large' It could be said that analysing transference is a treatment focused on the nature and extent of compliance itself.

In this regard, Figlio (1982) discusses that the relational context of psychotherapy has wider implications when trying to assess effectiveness and assessing evidence for it. Symptoms and their derivatives, syndromes, are in many cases socially constructed. The role of reconstruction in psychoanalytic technique, in investigating its technical value and in improving its therapeutic and conceptual basis, has been to some level ignored since Freud's death in 1939, although the use of it continued to exist in clinical practice. Blum

(1994) argues the relevance of reconstruction as a concept and as a specific technical intervention. He gives a comprehensive reassessment of reconstruction, and argues for the importance of applying and integrating it with other clinical and theoretical perspectives. Blum et al. (2003) further deliberated that almost every aspect of the problem of reconstruction is taken up, considered and elucidated from different angles. The patient affectively re-experiences the childhood trauma, and reworks the adaptation to it in the immediacy and safety of the analytic process and in the context provided by reconstruction. The adult neurosis takes account of later development, but is constructed on childhood psychopathology and vulnerabilities. A patient's conscious remembrance as reminiscence is not simply rejected as though it were completely inaccurate or irrelevant. The patient's conscious narration of past experiences and its gaps, inconsistencies, distortions and parable personal fables, provides the context for the analyst to understand better. Reconstruction then can start progresses in an analytic and historical context at deep level connecting the here and now and its relation to the past, come back to present.

Often most of these hypotheses only can be examined and validated in the form of working relations with patients and the use of transference, free associations and unconscious interpretations here and now in the process. If they can be conceptualised more precisely into specific concepts explaining sets of perceived pragmatic events and predicting consequences, they can be better evaluated analysts working either with individual or in group interactions for the achievement of genuine reliable authentic coherence. The validation in the clinical process, to a large extent, depends on being as clear and specific as possible about the hypotheses being put forward for validation. I am suggesting that while we make interpretations based on intuitive hypotheses arising from background orientations and collections of observed clinical facts of people background history, and transference here and now in the sessions – it is appropriate to also create appropriate analysis on patients' current experience and behaviour outside the sessions. For much of the time such inferences is more in the form of working interpretation and making hypotheses explaining connections between sets of events and predicting consequences.

In spite all of these, it is important to recognise that in some cases there is no important connection between childhood events and adult psychopathology and if memory cannot be trusted to construct a self-description, then as analysts we need to find ways to understand patients psychological difficulties as much as possible to begin with. In therapy we listen, and we focus on the here and now, on problem-solving, and on helping patients to find new strategies and ways of interacting with the important people in their lives – but we also have to give attention to the patient's presentation of their past and its effect on the present, without putting too much emphasis on this, at least at the beginning. By doing this, through the memories and associations the patient will come to explore the mysterious otherness of oneself which is the job of reconstruction.

In summary my focus in this chapter is on methodology of assessments I used for the psychoanalytic perspective for group interventions. Whether the reader agrees that psychoanalytic assessment and treatments as a discipline has the capacity for group and specifically working with people endured or exposed to severe trauma, will be, dependant upon their reading of the psychoanalytic foundations and developments and on the philosophy, which I briefly addressed in this chapter. I consider this method of group intervention to be empirical, involving the testing of hypotheses and supporting psychoanalytical theories. As analysts, one important issue that we always need to give attention to is that it is reality that we can on occasions get frustrated or angry with our patients, being attracted to them or repelled, fascinated, uninterested, fed up, bored to death by them. So, we need to accept while we are analysts, we are human, so we are subject to all the same feelings in relation to others, including people we work with. Our training of course helps us to keep our boundaries and distance, and to know ourselves well enough to minimise our countertransference and not acting out towards any of the above, preventing potential risks to patients and ourselves. While in our own analysis, supervisions and training we gain a good knowledge of ourselves, it is always possibility of an imperfection and not knowing especially when we are facing unfamiliar and challenging situations.

The psychoanalytic concept of countertransference was an early contribution to understanding these sorts of dilemmas within the analysts and patient dyad that I will address in more detail in another chapter. It refers to the analyst's feelings toward the patient, particularly those that may be unconscious and stem from unresolved relationship issues and childhood experiences. We are trained to reflect on our own feelings, work on our own unresolved issues, acquire supervision, read, think and reflect on concerning challenges in therapeutic encounters with each patient as a dyad relationship, indeed be honest to refer the patient elsewhere, if we are not able to work with before we may get to a place of compromising our professional integrity and responsibilities. It does not matter how well-meaning we are initially; if we are not aware of own capacity and personal vulnerabilities and the necessity of unbreakable boundaries between ourselves and those we set ourselves to serve; we can potentially fail to set firm boundaries in responding to the neediness, charm or attractiveness of our patients.

Chapter 3

Trauma

Trauma plays a significant role in the psychogenesis of violence. An awareness of the relationship between internal and external reality is not universal, and much depends on individual early developmental and life circumstances. Being exposed to and suffering multiple traumas during life, people generally can develop some psychological difficulties, and for refugees specifically these may adversely hinder the process of adaptation and integration in the host country. There is a need to consider this and search for appropriate support for the efficient integration of refugees and asylum seekers.

What is the cause of psychological trauma?

Experts in the field of health define psychological trauma in different ways. There are events that are outside the range of the individual's usual experience that can constitute exceptional mental and physical stressors. The range of events that are traumatic to an individual are as diverse as trauma responses. Traumatic events can be the most severe and extraordinary stressors that have low expectancy, probability and controllability, while regular life stressors, in different areas of human experience, are ordinary and have high expectancy, probability of happening and controllability. Emotional trauma can result from occurrences such as a car accident, break-up of a significant relationship, a humiliating or deeply disappointing experience with a loved one, the discovery of a life-threatening illness or disabling condition, natural disasters, rape, persecutions, torture and other violent in war and conflict events, as well as responses to chronic and repetitive experiences such as child abuse, neglect, warfare, urban violence, concentration camps, racism and prejudice, battering relationships, and enduring economic and social deprivation.

Traumatising events can have an acute emotional effect on individuals involved, even if the event did not cause physical injury or immediate psychological problems. The definition of what is psychologically traumatic, consequently is fairly broad, and includes responses to powerful occurrences. It is difficult to determine in general whether a particular event is traumatic

DOI: 10.4324/9781003401322-4

for everyone. Usually the intrusion of the past memories into present is one of the main problems confronting the person who has endured trauma. For the purpose of identifying effect of trauma and its adaptive symptoms, I learned it is useful to ask the patient what has happened rather than what is wrong.

The idea of a protective shield or layer which allows only tolerable quantities of excitations is important in coping mechanisms. In the process of initial meetings or assessments, I pay attention to identify vulnerability and resilience factors of the patient before and after enduring trauma. Stress can deregulate the nervous systems for a relatively short period of time, for a few days or weeks, before the nervous system calms down and reverts to a normal state of equilibrium. This return to normalcy often is not the case when one has been affected by traumatic events. One way to tell the difference between ordinary stress and emotional effect of trauma is by looking at how a disturbing event affects a person's relationships and overall functioning in life. We can hypothesise if one can communicate distress to people and can respond adequately and return to a state of equilibrium, we are in the realm of stress. But if we turn out to be distant in a state of active emotional intensity, we surely are experiencing an emotional trauma, though sometimes we may not be consciously aware of it.

The accumulation of non-traumatic stressors, sufferings, or dilemmas can create trauma like experience and can eventuate post-traumatic stress (PTS)-like symptoms (I prefer not to use disorder in my discussion and specifically within psychoanalytic approach). They can also add up to the real traumas and amplify their effects. Negative socio-cultural attitudes and non-supportive responses toward the traumatised individual can create the chain of post-trauma stressors which may cause secondary traumatisation.

Understanding trauma and particularly effects of external trauma inflicted to people is essential and imperative for running trauma group. It is therefore important that we looked at theory that provide us a means to control, stabilise and contain our own anxiety about what is observed and what can be expected on our patients' road to recovery.

Trauma renders people helpless, overwhelming their ordinary systems of care that allow them to have a sense of control, connection, and meaning. When the overwhelming force is that of other human beings the trauma is especially damaging as compared with when the force is found in nature. Herman (1992), in her book *Trauma and Recovery*, considers that a person's response to trauma is usually manifested in three symptom clusters. These symptoms reflect the fact that each component of the ordinary response to danger, having lost its utility, persists in an altered and exaggerated state long after the actual danger is over. The hyperarousal and the persistent expectation of danger can create an inability to sleep, relax, eat; emotional liability as the person is easily upset, frightened or angered, intolerance, anxiety attacks and dissociative symptoms. Also, re-experiencing, the deep-seated imprint of the traumatic event. There are intrusive images, thoughts, memories, nightmares, and flashbacks. Constraint and limitation of the numbing response of surrender, where there isn't little or no affect, the person can't feel, can't cry, and can't remember. There is an avoidance of anything associated with the memory of trauma or anything emotional or upsetting; an avoidance of social connections, places and things of former interest; an overall disinterest in life's events or in the future.

The core experiences of psychological trauma are disempowerment and disconnection from others. Therefore, recovery is based on empowerment and the creation of new connections with self, having a sense of self and in relation to other, the belief system and the view of the world. She offers a three-stage process of healing and recovery as a basic for a group or individuals comes to therapy with effected by trauma.

Single traumatic event and repeated or ongoing trauma

There is a distinction between single and repeated traumas. Single shocking events such as earthquakes, hurricanes, floods, volcanoes, plane crashes, chemical spills, nuclear failures, robbery, rape and homicide can certainly produce trauma reactions, but the traumatic experiences that result in the most serious mental health problems are usually prolonged and repeated, at times continued over years of a person's life.

The single unexpected direct trauma may cause typical symptoms of relentless flashback and persistent avoidance and increased arousal. It does not appear to produce massive denials, psychic numbing, self-anaesthesia, or a personality disorder that characterises the PTSD, though this type of trauma can impair some areas of psychological functioning. Complex traumas continuous and repetitive ordeals that gain prolonged appalling anticipation in one area of human functioning which can produce severe effects on mental health such as dissociation, somatisation, and depersonalisation. Such trauma creates defence mechanisms of repression, denial, dissociation, somatisation, self-anaesthesia, self-hypnosis, identification with the aggressor, and aggression against the self. The impairment in emotional processing includes the absence of feelings, a sense of constant anger and frustration, deep sadness and fear, which is quite common in refugees' experience. Protracted stressors, inflicted with intent by persons, are much more convoluted to tolerate than accidents or natural disasters. If harm was inflicted deliberately in the context of a relationship, the predicaments are greater than of an incident. In situations where the injury is caused deliberately in a relationship with a person on whom the injured party is dependent, mainly by a parent or caregiver in relation to the child, the effect can be horrendous. Sadistic abuses and interpersonal violence by caregiver/s as an eruption of passions in the severest forms are those inflicted deliberately. Premeditated cruelty can be more terrifying and more injurious than impulsive violence. Experiences of war or political violence are usually enormous in scale; they are brutal, repeated, extended and volatile. Moreover they are often compounded by witnessing life-threatening events, and possibly by doing violence to others and embracing the identity of an executioner. Other situations such as kidnapping, torture, rape, domestic violence usually associated with a longer period of helplessness, fear of injury or death. Witnessing someone else being beaten is stressful and the greater the attachment to the person, the greater the stress is. Watching violence directed towards a parents or caregiver is devastating for the child due to the fear of losing his/her primary source of security. Coercive power which has been used in prison, concentration camps and in some families has overwhelming and destructive effects on the receiver.

Specifics to refugee types of events the enduring effects of a past event such as torture or sexual assault whether in childhood or as an adult can lead to a change in the person's perception of self, others and of the world. One may lack the capacity to cope or build the capacity for altering beliefs about self and the world to the extreme, in order to feel in control. One may believe that all officials might be potential perpetuators or rapists and the world is not a safe place. It is also possible to fail to assimilate and alter external resources to match previous beliefs, and come to believe that for the reason that a bad thing happened to 'me', 'I' must be getting punished for something terrible 'I' did, because bad things only happen to bad people; believing that life is dangerous and that 'I' should always fear what could potentially happen. However, during the normal processing of a past trauma the goal is to accommodate the trauma into our life, which means altering our beliefs to incorporate the new information. If we lack this capacity then we develop negative beliefs which further the stressors. For example, a traumatised patient may start to believe that the world is not always a just and fair place but there are exceptions and 'I' am a bad person for being persecuted or having to leave as a result of war; and sometimes bad things happen to good people, and the world is not an unsafe and insecure place altogether. However, if this person has a reappearance of the symptoms, or there is a rational fear and intrusive thought such as the asylum application may be rejected and they might be return to the dangerous situation they have fled, fears and intrusions might be justified and therefore the progression for adjustment to the unpredictable might be challenging, but this is a normal reaction to an abnormal situation.

Diagnosis and treatments of war neurosis and post-traumatic stress

It started after the First World War and continued with the Second World War. Later in the 1980s numerous trauma treatment models were developed which were collectively referred to as 'trauma debriefing' models. One common belief in these models was to encourage the traumatised person to re-tell the trauma story in as much detail as possible. While this chapter does not present detailed discussion of these methods and their variations, and a critique of whether these are sufficient, in my view there is no convincing evidence yet as to whether trauma debriefing aids or hampers the traumatised person's psychological recovery. This approach if used out of context by a caring person, who wants to help but has no counselling or other mental health training and qualifications or skills, is potentially dangerous. There is a rising body of research and literature on identifying, diagnosing and treating psychological trauma and trauma-related ill health and also on culturally determined means of communicating psychological distress and articulating symptoms. This augmented focus is associated with the need to make available suitable services to a rapidly growing population of displaced peoples, immigrants and refugees deracinate in a global situation of armed conflict, which unfortunately shows no signs of ending or of lessening. The World Health Organization (1995) provides a table summarising 11 studies of post-traumatic stress disorder (PTSD) prevalence rates in different populations that have suffered natural or man-made disasters, war, torture or repression. The occurrence rates vary from a low of three and one-half per cent among flood victims in Puerto Rico and four per cent among refugees at a health-screening clinic in the United States, to 88 per cent in Laotian refugees attending an Indochinese mental health program in the United States. These wide-ranging differences can be attributed in part to diverse assessment methods, scales and interview programs and partly to differences between child and adult populations. However, it is generally accepted that some refugees who have experienced torture, are at particularly high risk for developing mental health problems. Another common finding noted in these studies is the high frequency of comorbid psychiatric conditions, namely major depression and anxiety.

A beneficial approach in assessing trauma related psychological problems to make no assumptions regarding patients' narratives and explanations, illness, expectations for treatment, but verify their descriptions and rationalisations explicitly with them. The underlying rationale is that all clinical encounters are in fact cross-cultural encounters and this is worth considering even when patient and analyst are from the same cultural background. For example, the question, 'What was the worst part of the traumatic experience for you?' can often generate very different and unexpected answers even among people who have experienced the same event, this clarifies that individuals being in the same event have not experienced the same trauma. Culture also shapes experience of trauma and may give the illusion of a common destiny that would press out varying individual providence, while different destinies are contingently related together, and indeed shapes the effects of trauma and its intensity. Therefore, it is important to be aware of how the individual's psyche may find hidden paths within the constraints imposed by culture. In some cultures, trauma recovery also involves witnessing, testimony and reparation. The experience of trauma and recovery is distinct from the narrative frames of Western societies, which are often linked to Christian accepted wisdom (conscience or unconscious) of catharsis, confession, reparation, and redemption. In some cultures, it is safe to speak out as one may have a belief system that social testimonies are needed before healing can occur.

It is important to recognise that there is also controversy about diagnosing social and political problems related to violence, war or poverty as psychological disorders. By giving a diagnosis of PTSD, social protest or suffering becomes medicalised and pathologises people, who are persecuted under a repressive regime or as a result of ethnic cleansing, or particular beliefs or principles. In some cultures, distress is commonly understood and expressed in terms of disruptions to the social and moral order and no particular attention is paid to internal emotions. There is a great overlap between mental health and trauma and we need more studies of people who have lived through war and other traumatic experiences to have more realistic expectations regarding trauma effects of over time. In some cases, people who have experienced and/or witnessed massive trauma have been able to have productive levels of functioning. Psychosocial interventions therefore should focus more on increasing the capacity, rather than on predictable symptoms, dispensation.

Post-traumatic stress disorder (PTSD), a medical model

The diagnosis of Posttraumatic Stress Disorder (309.81) in the fourth edition (revised) of the *Diagnostic and Statistical Manual of Mental Disorders* (*DSM-IV-TR*) (American Psychiatric Association, 2000, pp. 467–468). In the fifth edition (*DSM-5*) (American Psychiatric Association, 2013) it is not much different, but the Posttraumatic Diagnostic Scale and the new PTSD items in *DSM-5* introduce positive factor analysis for change of *DSM-IV-TR* as a better comparable model fits with refugee types of trauma. The new Cluster D symptoms showed relatively high sensitivity, specificity, positive predictive power, and negative predictive power. The *DSM-5* symptom structure in my view on medical model appears to be more appropriate pertinent to traumatised refugees. Negative alterations in cognitions and mood may be especially useful for psychiatrists and other clinicians, not only to determine the extent to which an individual refugee is likely to meet criteria for PTSD, but also in providing a more objectives clinical intervention beyond medications. The difference in the DSM-5 criteria for PTSD include first, direct or indirect exposure to a traumatic event, followed by symptoms, focusing in four main categories: (1) intrusion, (2) avoidance, (3) negative changes in thoughts and mood, and (4) changes in arousal and reactivity.

The essential feature of posttraumatic stress disorder mainly addressed in *DSM-IV* is the development of characteristic symptoms following exposure to an extreme traumatic stressor involving direct personal experiences of an event that involves actual or threat of death or serious injury, or other threat to one's physical integrity; or witnessing an event that involves death, injury or a threat to the physical integrity of another person; or learning about unexpected or violent death, serious harm, or threat of death or injury experienced by a family member or other close associate. The person's response to the event must involve intense fear, helplessness, or horror (or in children, the response must involve disorganised or agitated behaviour). The characteristic symptoms resulting from the exposure to the extreme trauma include persistent experiencing of the traumatic event. Persistent avoidance of stimuli associated with the trauma and numbing of general responsiveness; and persistent symptoms of increased arousal – the full symptom picture must be present for more than one month.

In ICD-10, the tenth edition of the International Classification of Diseases (F43.1) World Health Organization, 1992) PTSD is defined as a disorder that people may develop in response to one or more traumatic event(s) such as deliberate acts of interpersonal violence, severe accidents, disaster, or military action. The disorder can occur at any age, including during childhood.

The ICD-10 definition states that PTSD may develop after 'a stressful event or situation ... of an exceptionally threatening or catastrophic nature, which is likely to cause pervasive distress in almost anyone' (p. 147). Thus, PTSD would not be diagnosed after other upsetting situations that are described as 'traumatic' in everyday language, e.g., divorce, loss of a job, or failing an exam. In these cases, a diagnosis of adjustment disorder may be considered. DSM-IV highlights that a traumatic stressor usually involves a perceived threat to life (either one's own life or that of another person) or physical integrity, and intense fear, helplessness, or horror. Other emotional responses of trauma survivors with PTSD include guilt, shame, intense anger or emotional numbing. The validated diagnostic instruments and most randomised controlled treatment trials of PTSD mainly use the diagnostic criteria for PTSD defined in DSM-IV-TR.

People at risk for PTSD include:

- Victims of violent crime (e.g., physical and sexual assaults, sexual abuse, bombings, riots).
- Military, police, journalists, prison service, fire service, ambulance and emergency personnel, including those no longer in service.
- Victims of war, torture, state sanctioned violence, terrorism and refugees.
- Survivors of accidents and disaster.
- Women following traumatic childbirth
- Individuals diagnosed with a life-threatening illness.
- Children in an abusive environment.

Symptoms of PTSD

The most characteristic symptoms of PTSD are re-experiencing. PTSD sufferers involuntarily re-experience aspects of the traumatic event in a very
vivid and distressing way. This includes flashbacks in which the person acts
or feels as if the event were recurring; nightmares, and repetitive and distressing intrusive images or other sensory impressions from the event.
Reminders of the traumatic event arouse intense distress and/or physiological
reactions. Symptoms of hyperarousal include hypervigilance for threat,
exaggerated startle responses, irritability, and difficulty concentrating and
sleep problems as well as symptoms of emotional numbing. These include
inability to have any feelings, feeling detached from other people, giving up
previously significant activities, and amnesia for significant parts of the
events. Other associated symptoms including depression, generalised anxiety,
shame, guilt and reduced libido, which contribute to their distress and
impact on their functioning.

Whether or not people develop PTSD depends on their subjective perception of the traumatic event as well as the objective facts. For example, people
who are threatened with a replica gun and believe that they are about to be
shot, or people who only contract minor injuries during a road traffic accident but believe at the time that they are about to die may develop PTSD.
Furthermore, those at risk of PTSD do not only include those that are
directly affected by a horrific event, but also witnesses, perpetrators and
those who help PTSD sufferers (vicarious traumatisation).

Effects of PTS

PTS symptoms cause considerable distress and can significantly interfere
with social, educational and occupational functioning. It is not uncommon
for PTS sufferers to lose their jobs, either because re-experiencing symptoms,
sleep disturbances and concentration problems, unable to cope with reminders of the traumatic event at work. PTS has adverse effects on the sufferer's
social relationships, and social withdrawal, problems in the family and break-
up of significant relationships. People may also develop further, secondary
psychological disorders as complications of the PTS. The most common
complications are: substance use, depression, risk of suicide; anxiety, panic
attacks, which may lead to additional restrictions (for example, inability to
use public transport); somatisation; chronic pain; and poor general health.

Diagnostic criteria of PTSD in the ICD-10

In this chapter I give some detaild about DSM, it is important to do the
same with the ICD-10 diagnosis of PTSD that requires the following:

(A) The individual must have been exposed to a stressful event or situation of exceptionally threatening or catastrophic nature, which would be likely to cause pervasive distress in almost anyone.

(B) There must be persistent remembering or 'reliving' the stressor in intrusive 'flashbacks', vivid memories or recurring dreams, or in experiencing distress when exposed to circumstances resembling or associated with the stressor.

(C) The individual must exhibit an actual or preferred avoidance of circumstances resembling or associated with the stressor, which was not present before exposure to the stressor.

(D) Either of the following must be present:

  1 Inability to recall, either partially or completely, some important aspects of the period of exposure to the stressor

  2 Persistent symptoms of increased psychological sensitivity and arousal (not present before exposure to the stressor), shown by any two of the following:

    a Difficulty in falling or staying asleep
    b Irritability or outbursts of anger
    c Difficulty in concentrating
    d Hypervigilance
    e Exaggerated startle response.

(E) Criteria B, C, and D must all be met within six months of the stressful event or the end of a period of stress (delayed onset by more than six months is possible, but should be specified). The ICD-10 diagnosis does not require a minimum duration.

In contrast to ICD-10, a DSM-IV diagnosis of PTSD further requires that the symptoms have persisted for at least one month. In the first month after trauma, trauma survivors may be diagnosed as having acute stress disorder. In the DSM-IV characterised symptoms of PTSD and dissociative symptoms such as depersonalisation, derealisation and emotional numbing also highlighted. The most characteristic symptomatic indications of PTSD are re-experiencing associated symptoms including depression, generalised anxiety, shame, guilt and reduced libido, which both contribute to distress and impact on functioning. The DSM-IV diagnosis of PTSD is stricter in that and puts more emphasis on avoidance and emotional numbing symptoms. It requires a particular combination of symptoms (at least one re-experiencing symptom, three symptoms of avoidance and emotional numbing, and two hyperarousal symptoms). In addition, DSM-IV requires that the symptoms cause significant distress or interference with social or occupational functioning.

Research on PTSD

The example of main findings from the epidemiological research on PTSD are:

- The majority of people will experience at least one traumatic event in their lifetime (Kessler et al., 1995).
- Intentional acts of interpersonal violence, in particular sexual assault and combat are more likely to lead to PTSD than accidents or disasters (Kessler et al., 1995; Stein et al., 1989).
- Men tend to experience more traumatic events than women, but women experience higher impact events (i.e., those that are more likely to lead to PTSD; Kessler et al., 1995; Stein et al., 1997). In a large representative USA sample, Kessler et al. (1995) estimated a lifetime prevalence of PTSD of 7.8% (women: 10.4%; men: 5.0%). using DSM-IIIR criteria. Estimates for the 12-month prevalence range between 1.3% (Australia; Creamer et al., 2001) and 3.6 % (USA). Estimates for one-month prevalence range between 1.5% and 1.8 % using DSM-IV criteria (Stein et al., 1989; Andrews et al., 1990, and 3.4% using the less strict ICD-10 criteria (Andrews et al., 1990. PTSD remains common in later life but with the suggestion of a greater proportion of subsyndromal PTSD in the older age group.

Rape was associated with the highest PTSD rates in several studies. For example, 65% of the men and 46% of the women who had been raped met PTSD criteria in the Kessler et al. (1995) study. Other traumatic events associated with high PTSD rates included combat exposure, childhood neglect and physical abuse, sexual molestation; and for women only, physical attack and being threatened with a weapon, kidnapped or held hostage. Accidents, witnessing death or injury, and fire/natural disasters were associated with lower lifetime PTSD (Kessler et al., 1995).

Different types of traumatic events are associated with different PTSD rates. Rape was associated with the highest PTSD rates in several studies. For example, 65% of the men and 46% of the women who had been raped met PTSD criteria in the Kessler et al. (1995) study. Other traumatic events associated with high PTSD rates included combat exposure, childhood neglect and physical abuse, sexual molestation; and for women only, physical attack and being threatened with a weapon, kidnapping or being held hostage. Accidents, witnessing death or injury, and fire/natural disasters were associated with lower lifetime PTSD (Kessler et al., 1995).

Assessment instruments identified for PTSD

Validated structured clinical interviews that facilitate the diagnosis of PTSD used within the provision clinical services are not limited but mainly include are:

- Structured Clinical Interview DSM-IV.
- Psychometric properties of the Posttraumatic Stress Disorder Symptoms Scale Interview for DSM-5 (PSSI-5) (PSS-I; Foa et al., 2016).

All these instruments are based on the DSM-IV definition of PTSD.

There is a range of useful self-report instruments of PTSD symptoms, including:

- Impact of Event Scale (IES; Horowitz et al., 1979) and Impact of Event.
- Scale- Revised (IES-R; Weiss & Marmar, 1997).
- Post-traumatic Stress Diagnostic Scale (PDS; Foa et al., 1998).
- Davidson Trauma Scale (Davidson, 1996).

Clinical aspects of the diagnostic interview

When establishing the diagnosis of PTSD, it is important to bear in mind that PTSD sufferers find talking about the traumatic experience very upsetting. People may find it hard to disclose the exact nature of the event and their associated re-experiencing symptoms and feelings, and may initially not be able to talk about the most distressing aspects of their experience. This may particularly be the case for people who experienced the trauma many years ago or have a delayed onset of their symptoms.

The main presenting complaint of sufferers does not necessarily include intrusive memories of the traumatic event. Patients may present with depression and general anxiety, fear of leaving their home, somatic complaints, irritability, and inability to work or sleep problems. They may not relate their symptoms with the traumatic event, especially if significant time has elapsed since the event. Epidemiological research has shown that the diagnosis of PTSD is greatly underestimated if the interviewer does not directly ask about the occurrence of specific traumatic events. It is call to mind that checklists of common traumatic experiences and symptoms may be helpful for some patients who find it hard to name them.

The DSM-IV diagnostic category for PTSD is a widespread tool for measurement and comparison of symptoms, aiming toward diagnosis and, thus, treatment of this condition. Perhaps more than other psychiatric diagnoses, though, the concept of trauma necessitate a broader view to enable a methodical perceptive of the experience, even when it is observed in a bio-psycho-social formulation. This may be due in part to the exceptional cause effect nature of PTSD, where an event that threatens life or appendage is essential to the diagnosis. This aetiology creates an opening for interpretation and a need to search for the meaning that a traumatic event has on individual. Additionally, developmental process, psychological resilience and other social factors that protect people from developing PTSD must be explored to understand why large numbers of people who have in fact experienced trauma do not develop the illness as defined by the DSM-IV diagnostic category for PTSD classification. *DSM-IV* changed criterion A of PTSD by omitting the description of the stressor as 'outside the range of normal human experience'. Instead, criterion A now requires that the individual's experience in response to the stressor must include intense fear, helplessness or horror. This definition expands the type of traumatic events that qualify for PTSD to include violent, personal assault, motor vehicle accidents, natural or manmade disasters, learning about the sudden, unexpected death of a family member or a close friend, learning that one's child has a life-threatening disease, or being diagnosed with a life-threatening disease.

The defining characteristic of a traumatic stressor or of psychological trauma is the presence of an implicit or explicit life-threat and reactions that are extreme and generally negative. The development of PTSD may be only one of many related consequences of exposure to trauma. There are other stressor that can be considered, most of which reflect the effects of life-threat on biological, emotional, or cognitive functioning. Traumatic stress may thus be associated with unusual or unique endocrine changes, immune system changes, upset and distress, cognitive distortions, and existential anxiety. These changes may occur as a function of direct threat, as when one is diagnosed and treated for serious illness, or more indirectly, as a function of witnessing. For the most part they occur because of the life-threat involved, and this threat or its direct implications form the core of an emotional complex that appears to reason for restructure or change of one's perception of the world.

If the focus of threat to life is not based on a past event for patients but is based on the future, which is the case in many asylum seekers, the intrusions and re-experiencing symptoms that occur as part of posttraumatic stress syndromes may be of a different type than those experienced by individuals exposed to traditional traumas. The re-experiencing symptom act as a guidance of PTSD is totally stand on past trauma exposure, rather than future oriented events. Some asylum seekers who are seeking psychological help who are having intrusions that consist exclusively of the past event, may also have future orientated intrusions (e.g., will the Home Office accept my Asylum Application? Will my children progress with their education in this country? Will I see my hometown again in my life? Will I ever learn this language? Will I ever be able to work again? What will happen to me if they send me back? Will my children be provided for if I die? The list can go on). The only way to examine this empirically is to ask patients about the content of their intrusive thoughts, rather than make assumptions.

It seems to be too much emphasis and attention to medical model diagnosis of PTSD in refugee patients who may have endured or witnessed trauma and suffer acute stress symptoms. Qualitative analyses needed to determine the types of intrusive thoughts that refugee patients experience, and re-examine categorisations of psychological problems and whether these stressors are experiences as being future or past event oriented. Existing research examining PTSD across the diagnosis and treatment range for refugee patients has shown that the diagnosis is not straightforward in refugee patients, as there have not been clinical research to evaluate whether some intrusions are current and future oriented and is not belong to past. I am specifically thinking of the social circumstances an asylum seeker faces, such as uncertainty in immigration status, work, housing etc. In contrast to medicalised view I presented above, the literature on social suffering shed a better lights on human suffering. Kleinman et al. (1997) elaborate on traumatic experiences and human problems in a much more meaningful manner and allows for a more humanistic understanding of the challenges that we all face in our lives. Suffering is described by Kleinman and colleagues (ibid.) as a social experience that connects the moral, the political and the medical, including health and social policy. The social constructionist Burr, (2003) emphasis that there is not one correct or true way of viewing the world, rather there are many different realities all constructed within different contexts. It is important to address cognitive behaviour therapy (CBT) here as well.

Although there is evidence that differences exist in factual knowledge among all traditional practices, when it comes to psychoanalysis, a controlled randomised comparison study has not yet been conducted, to address this issue as principle. A comparison study of learning styles and attitudes to mental health, and an examination of performance change in patients from a traditional problem-based learning therapeutic approach and a psychoanalytic approach, seems to be a sensible study that could provide scientific evidence, combined with professional judgment. It can be hypothesised that if the psychoanalytic approach becomes part of the curriculum for mental health education, it could result in increased deep learning, which would enable more favourable attitudes to psychoanalysis that lead to long-term improvement in mental health service performances. The focus should be related to the use of deep and strategic learning intercultural approach, listening and respecting patients' narratives and their view, rather than traditional model of practice of ticking boxes. Patients in the long-term can become better-equipped problem solvers and self-directed learners; they may be better able to learn and recall information they have gained and internalised in therapy and are better able to integrate basic self-knowledge into the solutions to problems, towards integration.

Although some of these claims find theoretical support from the literature on the psychology of learning, to date there has been no review of the experimental evidence supporting the possible differences in patients' long-term learning that can be attributed to the success of one approach or another – and the differences in short term interventions and possible relapse. For example, currently there is no strong evidence of improvement in patients who drop out. Also, learning in therapy, the patient may initially have increased or reduced levels of learning due to trauma recall and possible increase in anxiety and depression, but may or may not foster, over periods up to several years, increased retention of self-knowledge. Moreover, CBT is designed to help solve problems in people's lives and intend to change people's thoughts, beliefs, attitudes and expectations, and how they act. This approach in my view may works well with young professionals coming from liberal family and not learned well to have and comply with boundaries – in a sense not experienced super-ego. In contrast, most of refugees who suffered state and political trauma, all their suffering may inflict by strong super-ego. In psychoanalytic interventions our focus is on these changes more deeply for patients.

To summarise, so far I argue that considering psychoanalytic practice offers a critical position from which the field has the ability to increase its effectiveness and relevance in working with people who suffer from complex psychological problems that are too often failed by other therapeutic methods conventionally accepted and practiced within mental health services. As with all methods, continued scrutiny will be essential to maintain the validity of psychoanalytic findings. Thus, as a psychoanalyst, like many of my colleagues globally, I know I must remain open to find a new ways to provide evidence that has the potential to falsify as well as adhere to strict methods of collecting and collating data for the purpose of increasing patient's strength and balanced and maintainable psychological recovery and growth. Establishing the significance intercultural approach within psychoanalytical framework have been fundamental key for improving the effectiveness of the psychoanalytic clinical interventions in my practice for almost four decades.

What so far trauma means

Trauma plays a significant role in the psychogenesis of violence. A normal awareness of the relationship between internal and external reality is not universal, but rather a developmental achievement (Fonagy & Target, 1996, 1997). Karen Horney (1945) discussions on inner conflicts. After suffering multiple traumas during their lives, people in general, will have some psychological difficulties, and for refugees specifically, these hinder the process of adaptation and integration in the host country. There is therefore a need to think about this and search for appropriate help for the efficient integration of refugees and asylum seekers. Erikson suggests 'man is the animal that has learned to survive "in a fashion," to multiply without food for the multitudes, to grow up healthy without reaching personal maturity, to live well but without purpose, to invent ingeniously without aim, and to kill grandiosely without need' (Erikson, 1964, p. 227).

The psychological intrusion of the activity altered condition of mind due to stimulation that is excessive in relation to the leniency and tolerance of the person psychical organisation mechanism. Whether it is a case of a single traumatic event creating strong emotion or of an accrual of stressful events each of which could be tolerated by the person at first, but in the process of the precept of consistence endurance is enfolded the mechanism of psychic organisations which the person become vulnerable powerless of discharging the excitation. This line with Laplanche and Pontalis (1964) focusing on Freud conceptualisation of this state of affairs in the 'Beyond the Pleasure Principle' (Freud, 1920), seeing it in terms of a basic uncomplicated relationship between an organism and its surroundings. They are suggesting that the 'living vesicle' is sheltered from external stimuli by a protective shield or layer which allows only tolerable quantities of excitation through. Due to this breach, the person will suffer trauma and 'the task of the apparatus at this juncture is to muster all its available forces so as to establish anticathexis, to immobilise the inflowing quantities of excitation and thus to permit the restoration of the necessary conditions for the functioning of the pleasure principle' (Laplanche & Pontalis, 1967).

What is the cause of psychological trauma?

Experts in the field of mental health define psychological trauma in different ways. There are events that are outside the range of the individual's usual experience that constitute exceptional mental and physical stressors. However, the ranges of events that are traumatic to the

Internal and external trauma

There are also fundamental differences between internal and external trauma. Trauma is an event which is almost impossible to forget and its endurance may result in some psychological trouble or psychological growth. Object relation theories is helpful to distinguish these differences and its consequences. The external characteristics of the potential traumatic event can start indirectly and become the most severe and direct trauma. Following Klein (1975) interest in the very earliest stages of the mind, Bion hypothesised that the first cognitive working of the mind entails a link between something innate (the organism itself) and something foreign (experience perceived in external reality; cited in Hinshelwood, 1999). So, trauma can be factitious and actual, and stimuli can be either internally induced or externally inflicted, by natural or manmade disaster.

Objective and subjective views of trauma

There are, in general, two components to a traumatic experience: the objective and the subjective. The subjective experience of the objective events constitutes the trauma. The more we feel and believe that we are endangered, the more traumatised we can become. It is our subjective experience and the level of strength and buoyancy we have that determines whether an event is traumatic and to what degree. Psychological trauma may be any type of event or encounter which causes an overwhelming emotion and a feeling of helplessness. There may or may not be physical harm. Psychological harm can result in physiological disturbances and create confusion between mind and body that plays a most important role in the long-term effects and presentation of trauma. Therefore trauma is distinct according to how we are experiencing it. It is not possible to make a general and comprehensive overview. The specific aspects of an event that are traumatic can vary from one individual to another.

Why can an event cause different responses in different people?

There are simple factors such as the severity of the event, the individual's ability to dissociate, strengths and weaknesses which is due to the early developmental process.The larger meaning an event represents to a person, the more traumatic effect it will have on one's psyche, which may not be straightforward. This also depends on numerous factors which influence person's personality structure, values and the way of thinking, level of resilience, coping mechanisms and support strategies such as availability, reaction and support from family, friends or professionals whose help one may seek. People can go through the same harmful event and some might be traumatised while others remain relatively unharmed or even become stronger as a result of the experience. People coping mechanisms and protective shield allows only tolerable quantities of excitations. This is important to vulnerability and resilience factors for people who have endured trauma in adult life.

Coping with trauma and stress

Stress can deregulate nervous systems for a relatively short period of time, for a few days or weeks, before the nervous system calms down and reverts to a normal state of equilibrium. This return to normalcy is often not the case when one has been affected by traumatic events. One way to tell the difference between ordinary stress and the emotional effect of trauma is by looking at the degree to which an upsetting event is remains affecting a person's life, relationships and overall functioning. If reason for distress can be communicated and be respond to adequately and be return to a state of equilibrium, one is in the realm of stress. But if one turns out to be distant, in a state of active emotional intensity, the person is experiencing an emotional trauma, though sometimes this may not be in conscious awareness of the level of distress one is experiencing.

The accumulation of non-traumatic stressors, sufferings, or dilemmas can create a trauma like experience and can produce effects similar to other types of trauma and eventuate with PTS symptom presentations. They can also add to the real traumas and amplify their effects. Any negative socio-cultural attitudes and non-supportive responses toward the traumatised individual can create a chain of post trauma stressors which may cause secondary trauma. This is relevance when considering the trauma experienced by refugees. As discussed before, there is a distinction between single and repeated traumas. Single shocking events such as earthquakes, hurricanes, floods, volcanoes, plane crashes, robbery, rape and homicide can produce trauma reactions, but the traumatic experiences that result in the most serious mental health problems are usually prolonged and repeated, and at times can continued over years of a person's life. The single unexpected direct trauma may cause typical symptoms of relentless flashbacks and persistent avoidance and increased arousal. It does not appear to strain the massive denials, psychic numbing, self-anaesthesia, or a personality disorder that characterised in the PTSD symptoms of medical diagnosis, though this type of trauma can indeed impair some areas of psychological functioning. In contrast complex traumas, which are continuous and repetitive ordeals that gain prolonged and appalling anticipation in one area of human functioning, produce the most severe effects on mental health. Such trauma creates enormous defence mechanisms of repression, denial, dissociation, somatisation, self-anaesthesia, depersonalisation, self-hypnosis, identification with the aggressor, and aggression against the self. The impairment in emotional processing includes the absence of feelings, a sense of constant anger and frustration, deep sadness and fear, which is all quite common in refugees' experience. Toleration of protracted stressors, inflicted with intent by persons, is much more complex than the toleration of accidents or natural disasters. If harm was inflicted deliberately in the context of a relationship, the predicament is greater than that of an accident. In situations where the injury is caused deliberately in a relationship by a person on whom the injured party is dependent, mainly by a parent or caregiver in relation to the child, the effect can be horrendous.

Disturbances of attachment

Attachment disturbances impact the shared affective exchange between parents or care givers with an infant and child, and companionship for an adult. It affects the feeling of warmth and connectedness for the adult and the feeling of security and trust for the child who depends on the attachment figure. Early childhood trauma that affects attachment includes abandonment, death of parent(s), and a parental affair or divorce. Loss of close significant others such as long-term child minder or care giver also can disturb the whole sequence of emotional development and can harvest an avoidant or muddled and confused object relation style. This can engender connection and relating and can leads to personality difficulties, detonate assumptions and viewpoints about self and objects, and impact on emotional as well as rational thinking and functioning in the area of object relations. The relevance of object relations theory I will discuss in more depth later.

The formation of a sense of identity, agency, and self-efficacy is a developmental milestone to adulthood with affirmative consequences on individual wellbeing. Self-sufficiency or development of positive identity builds emotional independence which leads to feelings of being competent, adequate and in control over self and in relation to others. Trauma such as sexual and physical abuse, domestic violence, rape, slavery, being a prisoner of war, torture, and genocide can disturb psychological connectedness and cause feelings of loss of self and helplessness in adulthood, and in childhood can disturb the development of a healthy object relation, autonomy and identity formation.

People interrelate within a set of connections that provide emotional, social, and material support as well as a sense of being socially entrenched, have a sense of belonging and meaning in life. There is also development of a system of accustomed social contingencies that are rooted psychologically and emotionally as the basis of feelings of safety, security, and belonging. Events that may threaten these associated and connected networks and well-established associations can be traumatic. Forced exile and displacements for refugees can mean the loss of connectedness by suspension.

Disturbances of social behaviour

Our social behaviour is usually motivated by the pursuit of our goals that are central to our perception, the value and component of our behaviour based in our evaluations of our prospective targets. Our failure to achieve a target that is perceived essential and possible can also be traumatic. So, in one hand it is possible that the effect of trauma may prevents one of achieving target, and also the failure to achieve the target may causes the trauma. Some traumatic events can affect more than one value processing subsystem. For instance incest can disturb both healthy attachment and autonomy, and genocide can disturb collective identity, interdependence and community subsystems, and demobilise one's psychological resources to respond, which can overrule all other sub-systems. These types of experience can shatter the schema, beliefs, assumptions, representations and judgments about the self and the view of the world, and about the efficacy of the existing value processing mechanisms that we possess.

Traumatic events therefore can adversely disturb the person automatic functions that execute the automatic activation of schema. They may be beyond the prevailing and surviving repertoire of schemata and representations of a person that direct the adaptive response to such events which may put a demand for novelty toward fresh quantity denomination processing structures. Moreover, as a result of the trauma a person can perform manners that do not match the personality and value system prior to enduring trauma. Paradoxical principles morality, committing decadent can develop in a person to survive which is possible to become excessive in the process beyond and against the person highly developed principles for order of moral goal; the domestic violence for instance by a person after torture. It represents one of the potential behavioural components of trauma response, and in my clinical work many refugees who suffered multiple traumas by persecutions, imprisonments, torture and human rights violations can find this pattern of paradoxical morality unmanageable.

Some of the common patterns of emotional trauma may result in compulsive behaviour patterns, self-destructive, uncontrollable reactive thoughts, an inability to make choices, dissociative symptoms by splitting off parts of the self, and the inability to maintain close relationships. One way to determine whether an psychological trauma has occurred, perhaps even early in life before language or conscious awareness were in place, is to look at the kinds of recurring problems one might be experiencing. These can serve as clues to an earlier situation that caused a deregulation in the structure or function of the mind/brain. Forward-looking neurological research is beginning to show to what degree trauma effects people on a biological and hormonal basis, as well as psychologically, cognitively and behaviourally. In traumatic experiences and interruptions of normal development in childhood, hypervigilance of individual autonomic structure is compounded and reinforced by significant changes in the brain. So, we can say that trauma is a complex combination of biological, psychological and social phenomena.

Over time, even without professional treatment, symptoms of an emotional trauma may subside and normal daily functioning slowly but surely returns. However, in some cases the symptoms do not go away, or they may appear to be gone but then surface again in another stressful situation. However, when a person's daily life functioning or life choices continue to be affected, then they may require expert help. There are common effects or conditions that may occur following a traumatic event. Sometimes these responses can be delayed for months or even years after the event. Often people do not associate their symptoms with the precipitating trauma. Symptoms of a typical, unresolved trauma can fit under:

- *Physical* – e.g. eating disturbances, sleep disturbances, sexual dysfunction, low energy, chronic unexplained pain.
- *Emotional* – e.g. depression, spontaneous crying, despair and hopelessness, anxiety, panic attacks, fearfulness, compulsive and obsessive behaviours, feeling out of control, irritability, anger and resentment, emotional numbness, withdrawal from normal routine and relationships.
- *Cognitive* – e.g. memory lapses especially about the trauma, difficulty making decisions, decreased ability to concentrate, and feeling distracted or disoriented.

What are the common reactions to trauma?

Most people who directly experience a major trauma have problems in the immediate aftermath. Some of the most common problems after a traumatic experience are avoidance of situations that resemble the initial event, flash-backs or re-experiencing the trauma, detachment, depression, guilt feelings, grief reactions, an altered sense of time, increased sensitivity or arousal such as hyper vigilance, jumpiness, overreactions including sudden unprovoked anger, an extreme anxiety and a sense of being on guard, obsessions with death, sleep disturbances such as insomnia or nightmares, emotional numb-ing, fear, relationship problems and substance misuse. Some of these are further detailed below:

- *Avoidance and numbness.* Avoidance is a way of managing trauma related pain. The most common is avoiding situations that are a reminder of the trauma, such as the place where it happened, or going out in the evening if the trauma occurred at night. An added way to reduce discomfort is to try to push away painful thoughts and feelings. This can lead to feelings of numbness, where people find it difficult to have frightening or enjoy-able and affectionate feelings. Sometimes painful thoughts or feelings may be so intense that the mind blocks them out altogether, and in some cases, people may not remember parts of the trauma (this will be referred to as repression in later chapters). Lacking feeling in the here and now, even when recalling the traumatic experiences a refugee patient may avoid thinking about the actual experience or anyone and anything associated with the trauma.
- *Fear and anxiety.* Anxiety is a common and natural response to a dan-gerous situation. For many it lasts long after the trauma ended. This occurs when views of the world and a sense of safety have changed. People may become anxious when they remember the event. Other things which may trigger or signal anxiety include a place, time, smell, noise, or situation that is associated with the trauma.
- *Re-experiencing the trauma/flashbacks.* Intrusive thoughts, flashbacks, sudden floods of emotion or images related to the traumatic event are common for people who have endured traumatic experiences. People may re-experience unwanted thoughts of the trauma and vivid images as if the trauma were occurring again here and now.
- *Nightmares.* Nightmares are common. These symptoms occur because a traumatic experience is so shocking and so different from everyday experiences that it cannot fit into the customary world. Thus, in order to understand what happened, the mind keeps bringing the memory back, as if to better digest it and fit it in.
- *Increased sensitivity.* Increased arousal is also a common response to trauma. This includes feeling jumpy, stressed out, agitated and shaky,

being easily startled, apprehensive and having difficulty with concentrating and sleeping. If unattended to, continuous arousal can lead to impatience, irritability and personality change. People who have been traumatised often see the world as filled with danger, so their bodies are on constant alert, always ready to respond immediately to any attack. This increased arousal is useful in truly dangerous situations, but it can become very uncomfortable when it continues for a long time. An additional reaction to threat that can occur after a traumatic event is to freeze up.

- *Anger*. Many people who have been traumatised feel angry and irritable. If they are not used to feeling angry this may seem scary. Some people may feel angry in view of the fact that they are feeling irritable so often without knowing the reason. Anger can also arise from a feeling that the world is not an adequate and fair place anymore or as a result of loss and multiple losses in refugee's life.
- *Guilt*. Trauma often leads to feelings of guilt and shame. Many people blame themselves for things they did or did not do to survive, or feel ashamed because during the trauma they acted in ways that they would not otherwise have done in ordinary circumstances. Feeling guilty in relation to the trauma means admitting liability for what has happened. While this may help a person feel somewhat more in control, if sustained for a long time it can also lead to feelings of helplessness and depression.
- *Grief and depression*. Grief and depression are also frequent reactions to trauma. These can include feeling down, miserable, hopeless or despondent, losing interest in people and activities, feeling that life is not worth living and having sleep disturbances. These feelings can lead to thoughts of wishing to be dead or having suicidal ideation. Because the trauma has changed so much of how a person sees the world and their self, it makes sense for them to feel sad and to grieve for what has been lost as the result of the trauma.
- *Low self-esteem*. Self-esteem, confidence, self-image often become negative after a traumatic event. Many people view themselves as a disapproving personality and view others more unenthusiastically and to develop an idea that the world is unsafe and no one can be trusted. These negative thoughts processed over and over again construct the feeling of having been changed entirely as a result of the trauma.
- *Problems in relationships*. Relationships with others can become tense and it may be difficult to be involved in intimate relationships. People may find it difficult to feel sexual or maintain intimate relationships. This is particularly the case for individuals who have been sexually assaulted where, in addition to their difficulties with trusting people, sex itself is perhaps a reminder of the trauma.
- *Substance misuse*. After traumatic experiences some people may become more intense users of alcohol or other substances to self-medicate which

can cause additional problems. The greater the stressor, the more potentially detrimental the effects of trauma are, and the greater the need of substance use may be. When betrayal and damage is inflicted by a loved one who they articulated as doing well, the kernel of lasting mistrust and fear are planted. Thus, the survivor of repetitive childhood abuse and neglect expects to be harmed in any relationship and may interact with helping professionals as though they have the intention of harming them as well. The coping responses to abuse and neglect are varied and complex; a frequently traumatised person may carry numerous psychological difficulties which may differ from others including substance dependence, personality disorders especially borderline, depression, anxiety, dissociative disorders, and eating disorders.

Unresolved trauma from childhood

Childhood trauma, starting when the individual's personality is forming, shapes one's perceptions and beliefs. Traumatic stress in childhood that influences the brain is usually caused by poor or inadequate relationships with a primary caregiver/s. Sources of this relational trauma include forced separation in early life from primary caregiver; chronic lack of attention of a caregiver to the child's attachment signals, or reasons such as physical or mental illness, depression or grief. Early life trauma may create weak defences and vulnerability for experiencing future traumatic responses. Childhood trauma can also cause the disruption of basic developmental tasks and can have deficits in abilities such as self-love and respect, seeing the world as a safe place, trusting others, organised thinking for decision-making and avoiding exploitation. Disruption of these tasks in childhood can result in adaptive behaviour, for example self-love and respect will be replace by low self-esteem and agitation, paranoia, a lack of organised thinking for decision making, or psychosis, self-harm, self-destructiveness and self-sabotage. Trauma experienced at early points in psychological development may severely compromise the survivor's core sense of self (Kohut & Wolf, 1978) and the capacity for secure object relations, as well as the 'sense of self' and therefore relational representation. As a result, the strong sense and fear of harm, of death and of terror take away the patient 'sense of self' and of 'psychic space' of thinking and can place it with irreparable psychic damage. The unhealthy dissociations therefore become the patient's frame of reference, so, the treatment such as trauma exposure or of fear-based PTSD of re-experiencing the trauma memories and associated emotions in a narrative-building and control-enhancing manner is not useful intervention and may not work at all. This is partly because the patients do not have enough psychic space and ability to associate with the self or other, indeed with the memory of trauma endured in a manageable way. So, therapeutic intervention needs to support the patient's capacities to diachronically (experiences relating to or involving the developmental process of early life, especially the learning of language and reflection through time) or synchronically (relating to ego development or lack of it, especially the use of language, as it exists) manage primitive affect and impulses. In spite of this, there seems to be too much emphasis and attention on diagnosis of PTSD in refugee patients who are sufferers of acute stress symptoms. Qualitative analyses are needed to determine the types of intrusive thoughts that refugee patients experience and re-examine categorisations of these experiences as being past event oriented. Existing research examining PTSD across the diagnosis and treatment range for refugee patients has shown that the diagnosis is not straightforward, as there has not been clinical research to evaluate whether some intrusive thoughts are future oriented and may not relates to past. The best way to examine this empirically in my view is to ask patients about the content of their intrusive thoughts, rather than making assumptions based on standardised assessment forms.

I will suggest intercultural psychoanalytic practice is best to work with people endured trauma including refugees. In psychoanalysis we as analysts use ourselves in the therapeutic relationship; this is based on a therapeutic alliance between patient and analyst, intended to serve the purposes of the patient breakthrough and recognitions of the effect of trauma. The relationship is central to the therapeutic intervention; and the analyst is a major contributor to successful outcomes. I place the emphasis on self-reflective practice, self-understanding, interpersonal encounters and sensitivity to countertransference and repair in maintaining an effective therapeutic alliance. By creating and maintaining an open distinctly formulated and secure therapeutic relationship, determining tenability for analyst and patient alike to focus upon complex interpersonal and intrapsychic issues at conscious, subconscious and unconscious levels and focus of transference and countertransference interaction of here and now in the consulting room.

I place arguments forward that psychoanalysis presents as an enquiry that is continuously developing through multi-dimensional evidence within the context of daily life. Thus, pragmatic 'facts' emerges through the patient-analyst dyad and involvements within transference-countertransference, not concrete and undependable; just as objectivity of the outer world succeeds and prevails a form of objectivity of the inner world that correspondingly can occur. I furthermore can argue that if the inner world can be conceived of as a source of objective data, then it has to be and can be testable. In order to test observations, analysts inevitably impact the results acquired which occurs in all therapeutic approaches. The psychoanalytic approach offers a way for analysts to support patients to build resilience that can potentially be sustained throughout their lives rather than merely addressing one emergent problem. To determine the extent to which psychoanalysis as psychological therapy has the capacity to foster more enduring resiliency and recovery in patients requires disciplined implementation of clinical monitoring and evaluation that can provide evidence of a better effectiveness. Undertaking such a study will serve the psychoanalytic field not as a corroboration of 'evidence' to support a pre-existing theory, but rather as a critical clinical examination that analyses and compares outcomes and methods cross-disciplinarily for the purpose of improving the sustainability and appropriateness of treatment for those suffering psychologically.

The countertransference feelings that arose in analysts within therapeutic dyad and the question of consistency in analysts' countertransference feelings is indication of the analyst's own personal feelings, its manner and approach that is important in working with the patient feelings. Analysts' feelings are usually different with different patients and over time of process of analysis with each patient. The consistency in feelings toward the individual patients is impossible while deviations from consistency and importance of identifying and distinguishing the different aspects of the countertransference which are imperative to be observed and monitored regularly for the best practice. A meaningful use of the countertransference concept is very much based on systematic monitoring, examining and identifying of intermittent and out of the ordinary patterns in the analyst's effect and response. My approach, and the one we use at the refugee therapy centre, is intercultural psychoanalysis that focuses on building intercultural competencies in clinical intervention, with a specific focus on trauma and in particular traumatic experience of refugees, asylum seekers and destitute. I will stress the importance of the analyst's role in providing a containing relationship in which the deficits resulting from earlier developmental of the patient can be restored in the present through therapeutic dialogue. My clinical works both with individual and with group will take into consideration the culture, issues of separation, loss and arrival in the place of refuge, the social and intrapsychic impact of racism, prejudice and discrimination, social and welfare matters and circumstances. Such practice requires not just thinking, but having sensitivity, responsibility, maturity and ability to tolerate ambiguity, sever vulnerability, anger, mistrust and uncertainty. Through the many facets of this approach, we can develop a therapeutic point of view that has its own internal coherence which reflects our personal style. This necessitates a commitment to sustaining and tolerating several views, even when these appear to be contradictory to our own, in an effort not to exclude and foreclose hastily on a patient particular presentations or point of view. These differing views is important and very helpful as it serves as a system of continuing self-analysis and self-supervision so any interpretation will be thoughtful, flexible and responsive to the particular needs and circumstances of that particular patient, at a particular time, in a particular context. Such an approach to working with refugees can serve as an underpinning for both individual and group psychotherapy. I think we as clinicians need to think of ourselves as student and are committed to making ourselves to continuous learning and evaluation both professionally and personally stimulating, thought-provoking and stimulating self-testing.

In many cases I have worked both individually and in the group for almost four decades in my profession the devastating effect of traumatic events on people is the disruption of the ordinary life. For refugees specifically this can includes being forced to leave their home country and have lost the opportunity to have ordinary life. Understanding both the inner and outer worlds of the individuals, and the ways in which the past affects the present is important factors within group interventions for refugees who have endured trauma. The way in which what happened to traumatised refugees in the past is connected to how person associate and correlated past experiences and how can communicate and give an account of life stories and its effect in the present life. Furthermore, how becoming a refugee and how the trauma associated can be related to the person earlier developmental incidents the person was subjected to and lived through. The observation and conception that people have of their experience therefore is a central dynamic in the way in which people can handle the traumatic experiences, which is a process that could contribute to either gap in psyche or in creating strength and more psychic space. The ways in which a refugee patient can relates to past stories in the present is a function of the interplay of these components. The countless ways in which some refugees experienced physical and psychic invasion, is made all the more moving by the accompanying description of the capacity for creating a psychic space. The creation of this space, in which people are enabled to regulate their experiences in some way, either in fantasy or by action will be helpful to move on. The ability to create a space for thinking can be seen as linked to the quality of internal object representations, indeed to external events and opportunities. Winnicott's idea of potential space has understandable associations to the formulation of traumatised refugees and understanding the need for creating a psychic space. 'The potential space between individual and society depends on experience which leads to trust. ... exploitation of this area leads to a pathological condition in which the individual is cluttered up with persecutory elements' (Winnicott, 1970, p. 103). He says 'By creative living I mean not getting killed or annihilated all the time by compliance or by reacting to the world that impinges; I mean seeing everything afresh all the time. I refer to apperception as opposed to perception' (Winnicott, 1970, p. 41).

This space is the creation of this space that allows healthy dissociation, a defence mechanism which can foster strength and resilience. This is significant in both early developments as well as in later life when working with refugee. The effect of trauma, irrespective of previous personality structures, by and large influences people and their capacity to express painful events. It is an important factor in the way in which people recount their life histories. The ways in which effects are regulated during recall are related to narrative according to whether the traumatic association is direct or dominated by generational relation or not. This is not always an either/or question, as both healthy and unhealthy forms of association can be present at different times. This is a dynamic balance, which can be influenced by ongoing events (positive or negative) in individual life. I am hypothesising that some of the mechanisms of defence have curious idiosyncratic functions or we can say malfunctions. It seems less likely, for example, that someone would be filled with a sense of adventure and enthusiasm while peering out with wild animals as part of torture. Many other examples I can cite here from narratives of patients where people prior to seek refuge in a safer environments and become refugee have been endured. The concept of resilience adopted by many endured those atrocities as strategies should not overlook. It is important to bear in mind that the fact that many did not collapsed doesn't mean they have not been deeply affected. Regardless of how well they may have been able to recompense and counterbalance the movement from isolation and helplessness to connection with life, self and others are vitally important to be addressed in therapy when people decide to seek therapeutic help. I observed over and over many people seeking therapy themselves have some support networks around helping them to cope but still suffering in silence. Over and over I pleasantly surprised by some patients ability to have insights and great ability to be creative, intelligent, have sense of humour and are ambitions despite the experience of trauma.

Cross-generational transmission of trauma

Traumas are transmitted between different persons or generations with different mechanisms, such as symbiosis, empathy, attachment, enmeshment, personal or collective identification, projective identification, introjections, dependency, co-dependency, interdependency, parenting, compensation and acculturation. Individuals coexist in a system or network of intertwined relationships that transmit the effects of different significant events. An example is shared psychotic disorder; the development of a delusion in a person in the context of a close relationship with another person(s) who has an already established delusion (*DSM-IV*, 297.3). Traumas can have similar effects on people in relationships, or with strong collective identity, even if they did not suffer the trauma themselves. In this context, trauma can happen not only to one person, but also to a social unit, to a community, or sometimes to a whole society, such as genocide, civil war or ethnic cleansing.

This is important in our work within the group or when we are helping family. The transmission of trauma can happen from one person to another or to a connected group who has been affected by trauma and collectively may have lost their healthy defences and coping mechanisms. There are also indirect traumas and their effects which can transmit within a family system across generations, such as domestic or other type of violence, physical abuse, and incest. The intergenerational continuity of those family patterns is often expressed by young children becoming violent and perpetrators, or colluding with the victim role, repeating the intergenerational cycle of victim and perpetrator of violence. However, the transmission of trauma does not automatically occur for the same reason as an extreme traumatic event may not necessarily result in post trauma symptoms in all people to the same level.

Working with group I find attention to projective identification is helpful as a possible mechanism that can facilitate the transmission of unresolved traumatic experiences. Projective identification as we know it in the context of parent-child relationships involves the parent's recruitment of the child to perform a particular role for the parent's externalised unconscious phantasies. A child in the parent's projective fantasies may leads to a collapse of the Winnicott (1971) potential space within the parent–child relationship that allows the development of child's self-sufficiency and autonomy, though again, this transmission is not automatic.

Collective cross-generational trauma transmission is a complex trauma, as it is inflicted on a group of people that have particular group identity or affiliation to a collective culture such as ethnicity, colour, national origin, religion and political beliefs. Historical information prior to traumatisation and the intensity of traumatic exposure and its effects are important. Historical trauma can predispose the individual to meagrely respond to later traumas in life. Additionally there is the multigenerational transmission of political or structural violence resulting in extreme social disparities created by generating deprived social structures. The effects of deprivation by poverty experienced by people, of basic right in the country of origin, citizenship and immigration status in the new society that all may cause further trauma and lead to demoralisation and socioeconomic disadvantage in the new society where people seek refuge. Poverty may also halt intellectual development and cause educational deprivation for many refugee and asylum seekers, especially children and young people, even for those who have no apparent biological restrictions to learning. The direct and indirect cross-generational consequences of structural violation of basic human rights can be devastating and enduring to anyone. These types of ongoing traumatic conditions are the type which can, and in many cases will, transmit across generations.

Chapter 4

Repression and dissociation

The goal of this chapter is to determine the occurrence of various dissociative phenomena in patients who endured external trauma, and to discuss how, if these patients had a satisfactory early environment in the process of developments, even with horrific atrocity, they may have ability to tolerate and bear the pain by dissociating from memory of external trauma in adult life in a healthy and manageable way. Managing to survive atrocities that they have been endured and carry on with the day-to-day life requires strength and resilience. I have written on the resilience and healthy dissociations widly emphasising people with capacity for this type of dissociation is dependent on the early good environment and formation of resilient personality. In contrast those with unhealthy early life who are later affected by external trauma there may be levels of depersonalisation, derealisation, identity confusion, perversion, identity alteration, psychosomatic presentations and psychoses. This is vitally important from the initial assessments for group participants. Individuals with acute mental decompensation and compartmentalisation with certain thoughts, emotions, sensations the disturb memories are compartmentalised because it is too overwhelming for the person conscious mind to integrate. So, the person subconscious strategy for managing powerful negative emotions is splitting and dissociating from unbearable thoughts, emotions, sensations and memories from the integrated ego.

Psychic trauma is a situation in which the ego is overwhelmed and flooded by stimuli in a dangerous situation springing from within or without facing internal or external danger. In addition to the immediate traumatic situation or loss, and if not attended, persistent patterns of emotional turmoil can continue. The ego than can be reduced to primitive levels of cognition in dealing with aftermath of traumatic event which can be numbing, rages, outbursts of anger and violent behaviour and with freezing or disorganised frantic mobility. The over stimulation of affect often can be too powerful for the person ego to tolerate and worked with in an adaptive way. Freud (1926) placed emphasis on the traumatic state as one of psychic helplessness, quite different from that of merely anticipating danger. The symptoms can include

DOI: 10.4324/9781003401322-5

excessive, inhibited, intrusive or avoidant reactions, as well as a tendency towards repetition compulsion of the trauma, thought, feelings, and behaviour. Intrusive aspects include flashbacks, preoccupied fantasising, nightmares, somatic reactions, hyper-arousal and vigilance. Startle reactions are common as well as avoidance of situations resembling the trauma. Particularly regression and fixation to the traumatic situation can lead to developmental inhibition intrusions or interferences. Some people can experience a type of dissociation in which the traumatic experience or traumatic loss remains split off from total consciousness, the ego therefore becoming split from the object world. Loss of job and income can lead to economic deprivation or change in living situations while loss of loved one may lead to powerlessness and vulnerability intense negativity hopelessness. In the long term, if adequate mourning and adjustment cannot be brought about, pathological defence mechanisms such as denial, projection, or dissociation, or various forms of regressive behaviour can develop.

Here I bring a brief vignette of one of the group participants in a session who presented her issue with her line manager. She expressed her anger and frustration with her boss, saying in some instances the expression of her boss is irritating and she feels that she is victimised by her boss, and the system allowed this because of systemic prejudice and discrimination, if not conscious racism. She explained this ongoing situation causing much devastation and destruction on daily bases that she can feel is affecting her personal life, affecting her partner and their children too. She said her family living with a fear of her retaliation and this is unnecessary additional burden her partner and children are also often distressed and troubled.

If the assumption of dissociation being the disruption of the usually integrated functions of consciousness, memory, identity, or sensitivity to the environment, then how is it that through the act of dissociation some people survive massive trauma and human right violations? And what is missing in the people like the above patients who is not able to dear with sressers. An important consideration is the fact that when working with these types of patients, analysts need to be resilient. That being so, how we may successfully monitor our ability or lack of it? And, whether all types of therapeutic approach need to be aware not only of what patients bring, but also what analysts may introject or unconsciously bring and project to patients? It is reasonable to assume that if one has the opportunity to build a healthy attachment in early life, one become able to find a balance for living with psychological strength and resiliency.

In the chapter on trauma, I discussed in details but I feel it is important to address it briefly here what in psychiatry, dissociative disorders are. Four types of dissociative phenomena are described in *DSM-IV* as an acute or gradual, transient or persistent, disruption of consciousness, perception, memory or awareness; it is not associated with physical disease or organic brain dysfunction, and there is a miscellaneous fifth group. The distinction between these types may be blurred, particularly when patients exhibit symptoms from more than one type.

If the focus of threat to life is not based on a past event for patients but is based on the future, which is the case with many asylum seekers, the intrusions and re-experiencing symptoms that occur as part of posttraumatic stress syndromes may be of a different type than those experienced by individuals exposed to traditional traumas. The re-experiencing symptom acts as a guidance of PTSD is based totally on past trauma exposure, rather than future oriented events. Some asylum seekers who are seeking psychological help who are having intrusions that consist exclusively of the past event, may also have future orientated intrusions (e.g. Will the Home Office accept my Asylum Application? Will my children progress with their education in this country? Will I see my home town again in my life? Will I ever learn this language? Will I ever be able to work again? What will happen to me if they send me back? Will my children be provided for if I die? The list can go on and on). The only way to examine this empirically is to ask patients about the content of their intrusive thoughts, rather than make assumptions.

There seems to be too much emphasis and attention on diagnosis of PTSD in refugee patients who are sufferers of acute stress symptoms, including the dissociative disorder. Qualitative analyses needs to determine the types of intrusive thoughts that refugee patients experience, and re-examine categorisations of these experiences as being future or past event oriented. Existing research examining PTSD across the diagnosis and treatment range for refugee patients has shown that the diagnosis is not straightforward in refugee patients, as there have not been clinical research to evaluate whether some intrusions are future oriented and do not belong to past. There is also need to think and where possible do some research to explore whether all dissociations are mental illness or it is psychological strength to deal with aftermath of trauma.

A new way of thinking and working needed to be instigated for the provision of appropriate help for mental health in refugees. The intrusive thoughts possibly are both focused on the discrete past event and possible future oriented events. Such knowledge, understanding and developments may bring to light tangible evidence that the rates and patterns of unpleasant or traumatic experience are not as different across stressors in humans and refugee types of trauma may have another angular of experience of external trauma. Conceptualising post-trauma syndromes that may be characteristic of and specific to refugee patients is important, and could yield useful information about pre, post and future impact, the coping structure, resilience, the ability to adjust, and the management of health problems.

In contrast to a medicalised view, as part of the literature on social suffering, Kleinman's (1997) elaborates on traumatic experiences and human problems in a much more meaningful manner and allows for a more humanistic understanding of the challenges that we all face in our lives. He described suffering as a social experience that connects with our moral, political and social being as well as the treatment approach including medical model in health and social policy. The social constructionist, Burr (2003) emphasises that there is not one correct or true way of viewing the world, rather there are many different realities all constructed within different contexts.

In my view a healthy dissociations is a normal and an adaptive defence used to cope with overwhelming psychic pains as the result of trauma. It is commonly encountered during and after external trauma such as non-combatant citizen disasters, criminal assault, sudden loss, torture and war. In typical dissociation, the individual perception of the traumatic experience is temporarily troubled and may be deadened or dispelled from consciousness. This type of dissociation prevents other fundamental psychological functions from being overwhelmed by the traumatic experience. The capacity to dissociate, as evidenced by susceptibility to hypnosis, is not uncommon. However, it is unclear whether pathologic dissociation is an extreme or more enduring form of dissociation. I think post traumatic dissociation is an alteration in consciousness and awareness of the context of a traumatic experience.

It is possible to say that dissociation is separation of and or splitting off an intrapsychic defensive process, which operates automatically and unconsciously. Through its operation, emotional significance and affect are separated and detached from an idea, situation, or object. It is an unconscious process by which a group of mental processes is separated from the rest of the thought processes, becoming an independent functioning of mind which separates the affect with use of cognition in order to survive the unexpected external trauma. A state of mind in which some experience and memory of that particular experience will be separated from the rest of one's being and the ordinary personality and functions prior to the trauma and will function independently – this very act of dissociation is resilience which keep the personality intact by separating the experience of trauma which one cannot handle without feeling the psychological effects.

Janet (1907) created the term splitting in his book *L'Automatisme psychologique*, explaining it as a defensive mechanism employed in response to psychological trauma. He considered dissociation an effective defence mechanism that protects the individual psychologically from the impact of overwhelming traumatic events.

Freud (1919a) suggested that the notion of trauma fits into an economic perspective – that is an experience which within a short period of time presents the mind with an increase of stimulus too powerful to be dealt with or worked off in the normal way that may result in permanent disturbances of the manner in which the energy operates. Freud (1917) devised the term 'repression' to account for a patient's resistance to improvement. He used the term 'repression' both loosely to mean any ego defence (Freud, 1906), and specifically refers to the defence in which the idea is pushed into unconsciousness and so to be forgotten. He indicated that the associated effect of such an experience however, will remains in consciousness; and that the conscious ego which turn away undesirable thoughts and memories to the realm of the unconscious, is the way of surviving unacceptable material. Freud (1915) described a precursor of repression proper; and referred to trauma (Freud, 1920) as the cause of the mental organisation. He subsequently (Freud, 1923) invoked the super-ego as an additional agent to secure the repression of id material by the ego, and to inhibit part of the self – the id, by another – the superego. So, repression from his point of view is an active process and the model depends on a flat split between consciousness and unconsciousness. The theories of resistance and of repression, of the unconscious, of the aetiological significance of sexual life and of the importance of infantile experiences – these form the principal constituents of the theoretical structure of psychoanalysis are all related to internal trauma, conflicts and possible splits to contain and balance one's wish, will and desire.

Freud (1917a) also suggests that the very act of entering into civilised society entails the repression of various archaic primitive desires. His model of psychosexual development includes going beyond the previous 'love-objects' or 'object-cathexes' that are tied to earlier sexual phases; the oral and the anal-sadistic. Consequently, even well-adjusted individuals still betray the insistent force of those earlier desires through dreams, literature, or slips of tongue, hence the return of the repressed. In not well-adjusted individuals, who remain fixated on earlier libido objects or who are driven to abnormal reaction formation or substitute formations, two possibilities exist:

- perversion, in which case the individual completely accepts and pursues his or her desire for alternative objects and situations of sadomasochists; or
- neurosis, in which case the individual's prohibited desires may still be functioning but some repression is forcing the repudiated libidinal trends to get their way.

According to Freud (1915a, 1915b, 1915c), repression is a normal part of human development; indeed, the analysis of dreams, literature, jokes, and slips of tongue illustrates the routine that our desires continue to find outlet. However, when we are faced with obstacles to satisfaction of our libido's cathexis, or experience traumatic events, or when we remain fixated on earlier phases of our development, the conflict between the libido and the ego or between the ego and the superego can lead to alternative sexual discharges. The source of our sexual discharges is the libido which seeks to cathect or place a charge on first one's own bodily parts e.g. the lips and mouth in the oral phase and then external objects the breast and then the mother in the oral phase that Freud termed 'object-libido' which can get caught up in the ego and leads to narcissism, so, a normal part of psychosexual development therefore is the overcoming of early childhood narcissism. Freud's in his concept of repression and his theory of the unconscious fails to examine how people actually repress shameful thoughts. This is clear in some of Freud's classic case histories such as 'Dora' and the 'Rat Man' and the importance of small words in speech. Freudian repression offers insights on the use of language and discourse.

Although they differed significantly the fundamental common ground between Freud (1895a) and Janet (1907) was their interest in deeper, explanatory theories of hysteria and of the nature of mind. Their main difference is in their methods – eliciting unconscious reminiscences (Freud, 1895a), as opposed to suggestion or persuasion Janet (1907), as well as the origin of the unconscious (Freud) or the subconscious (Janet). Janet thought that, under stress, parts of the conscious mind became severed from the rest of consciousness (dissociation), while Freud described an active process of repression of certain contents of the mind, due to traumatic experiences in the past.

Dissociation is a better term for repression as it refers to those discontinuities of the brain, the disconnections of mind that we all harbour without direct awareness which let us to step aside, split off from our own knowledge, behaviour, emotions, and body sensations, and indeed our self-control, identity, and memory. Generally speaking splitting or disassociation involves different characteristics.

It is important to say that psychoanalytic writings at time regarded in opposition to trauma-based notions of human psychopathology. However, the psychoanalytic contribution and its emphasis on unconscious conflict and meaning is for the most part excluded from the discourse on dissociation, often resulting in a mechanic conceptualisation of trauma. But, the phenomenon of dissociation has been fundamental concept in the formation and development of interpersonal psychoanalysis (Sullivan, 1953) as well as the development of object relation theories (Winnicott, 1958a, 1965, 1971; Fairbairn, 1929b, 1954). Long before these developments, Breuer and Freud (1895) recognised dissociation as the central mechanism of hysterical symptoms as the result of a traumatic event that affected the brain's ability to process emotions. Since then, researchers studied the impact of trauma and the phenomenon of dissociation. Dissociation, or the splitting off of traumatic affect from conscious awareness, has been linked as a response to every type of traumatic experience.

Dissociation is posited as a form of psychical organisation in which psychical conflicts and threats to self-preservation are regulated on the mind and can be considered as a mechanism of de-repression when mind cannot coop with repression anymore. The dissociative communication is not necessary emblematic disposition but make use of a warning sign that augment to pseudo integration of psychological being rather than true personality integration. So, this can be considered as the foundation of the phenomenon of false self that may be observed in refugee patients. In this type of dissociation, the person skilfully creates an obscured line of defence the effect of which is to construct a narcissistic field of omnipotent constructions. So, the traumatised refugee may transform the experience and suspended beyond their conscious mind. It involves alterations in consciousness; as the person becomes aware of being in a state of ailment and may seeks help. This types of splitting off and dissociation can be measured as a normal phenomenon, potentially occurring as the result of external trauma and can be understood as more extreme and uncontrolled eruptions of these normal phenomena, often elicited in the face of traumatic stress. In my work with refugee patients I witness over and over how individuals seem to have an unusual capacity to control both mental functions, such as perception, memory, and attention, and somatic functions, especially in certain systems available to awareness and to reflect not so much being in or out of the conscious state on mind. For example, if an individual is taught to obstruct perception of a stimulus using compelling hallucination, changes can be observed in response to those stimuli which help the patient to learn to increase or decrease the flow to the manageable thinking. The less structured dissociative phenomena seem to provide enhanced access to control systems that interconnect the mind.

Base of such reasoning, dissociation can be considered as the structure of psyche that separates the opposing psychological tension as a natural necessity for consciousness to operate in way not to be burdened or obstructed by the demands of its opposite. In particular, the phenomena of double consciousness, split personality, or a plurality of personalities in individual that cannot appear in a usual circumstances. An individual's character-splitting is by no means impossibility, therefore, fully justified to argue there is possible for therapists to treat dissociation.

There is always dialectic between binary and dualistic selves in terms of autonomy and connection. People need to function psychologically in corrupt and devious environment they face; sometimes painful and against common humanity – but it is the real external reality. In these types of environment, although trauma inflicted beyond ones control, people need to keep their prior self in order to continue to see themselves as human. Thus, the self had to be both autonomous and connected to the prior self that gave rise to what the self come after endurance of trauma, to continue basic functionally. The splitting off the endured part and disassociate with that part in order to survive is the principles that help the self to succeed continuing to carry on, because it is inclusive and could connect with the entire environment, the aforementioned rendered coherent, and gave form to, various themes and possible mechanisms without falling apart.

This type of splitting and dissociation has a life-death dimension in which the self may perceive by the perpetrator as a form of psychological survival in a death-dominated environment. In other words, people can have the paradox of a killing self being created on behalf of what one perceives as one's own healing and surviving. Consequently, one function of splitting or disassociation is likely to be avoidance. In such state of mind the other disassociated self can be the one performing fraudulent but successful work of continue with the life without the total psychological collapse. This may involves both an unconscious dimension taking place largely outside of awareness and a significant change in righteous conscious awareness and decision making.

These characteristics construct and encompass what psychologically goes on in this type of division of mind and patterns of disassociating. The principle differentiation between disassociation from the traditional psycho-analytic concept of splitting is that the latter term has had several meanings but tends to suggest a holding off a part of the self, thus, the split off element ceases to respond to the environment or in some way probabilities to become at odds with the remainder of the self. This type of split is similar to what both Janet (1907) and Freud (1895a) originally called dissociation. In regard to persistent forms of how to explain the autonomy of that separated part of the self-confusion greater than usual, it is important to observe and identify what splits part in splitting in the psyche of a refugee patient who have endured trauma is dissociating in particular group session, why and whether an interpretations is appropriate there and then, or it is better to keep note and come back to it. Splitting or dissociating can thus denote something about psyche of a refugee patient who endured external trauma in the group, it is possible to be guilt, shame, embarrassments or lack of trust, indeed lack of consciousness with right vocabulary. In such situation the patient cognitive unconscious contains material that would be deeply disturbing if it did rise to consciousness without the appropriate space to working trough. Learning and understanding dynamics in the groups and after thoughtful concentrations and in consultation and discussion with colleagues, I increased the time of sessions from one and half hour to two to have space for one or possibly two participants who want to presents something painful and unbearable in the group. I consult this with one group first. The idea was welcomed. I had to think how we can set boundaries within this particular development. It was decided that in the beginning of each sessions people need more space will say so and group will make decision if more than one person needed space. This method not just helped those vulnerable at particular time but amazingly developed deep care and trust between participants. I practiced this only with one group first for 6 months, and then proposed it to my other groups, indeed proposed it to other colleagues running different groups at the Refugee Therapy Centre.

we know dissociative mind can overwhelms the suffering and disturbance of everyday life. These types of group interventions that is relationally structured with strategy and agreed boundaries, I find to be helpful for patients anxiety, confusion, splitting and anger. Thus feeling mostly arises out of unconscious and uncontrolled mind, to allow interaction even frightening, but still urgently needed connections with the self and others to survive. The dissociated self-states in my clinical work with refugee patients are among other trauma stress related clinical presentation that I work with as the ordinary everyday work including patients' expression of dreams, projective identifications, and enactments. By expressing these, I am not denying or ruling out that the pathological dissociation is possible to result when the psyche is overwhelmed by trauma and signals the collapse of relationality.

Clinical phenomena associated with splitting and disassociating I chosen to work with my understanding of relational model of psychoanalysis. I observed dissociation almost in all patients, so, relational focus interpretations I find helpful in alternating dissociated part of self that develops along an alignment of relational trauma.

In conclusion for refugees and others who endure sadistic and violent abuse and human rights violations in many levels, a healthy dissociation provides a means to sanity and survival. These mean splitting off their sentiments, permitting the compartmentalisation of experience, to keep going without psychological collapses. It is a motivated not forgetting but not remembering that provides temporary protection from the stress of horrific experiences, a manifestation in an effort to cope with persisted traumatic demands that contains the experience and memory of massive trauma and paradoxical realities which may engender a dissociating – it is not out of mind, but it is in parallel mind to keep the mind going. In including conflict, unconscious intention and personal meaning in understanding the kind of dissociation it is possible to see patterns of affect regulation and dominant object-relational strategies that can be recognised and worked through in discourse of therapeutic encounters, mainly through narrative, dreams and unconscious, indeed transference and countertransference interpretations.

In my view, dissociation is one of the most important concepts and perceptions in working with refugees and others who endured external trauma such as persecutions, imprisonments, captivity, torture, war and natural disasters. It is a function of the mind to push certain experiences into some inaccessible corner of the unconscious that later can emerge into subconscious and consciousness.

Chapter 5

Principles of psychoanalysis in relation to trauma

Sigmund Freud (1856–1939) made us aware of two powerful forces and their demands on us. Back when everyone believed people were basically rational, he showed how much of our behaviour was based on biology. When everyone conceived of people as individually responsible for their actions, he showed the impact of society. When everyone thought of male and female as roles determined by nature or God, he showed how much they depended on family dynamics.

Second is the basic theory, going back to Breuer, of certain neurotic symptoms as caused by psychological traumas. Although most theorists no longer believe that all neurosis can be so explained or that it is necessary to relive the trauma to get better, it has become a common understanding that a childhood full of neglect, abuse, and tragedy tends to lead to an unhappy adult.

Third is the idea of ego defences. Even if you are uncomfortable with Freud's idea of the unconscious, it is clear that we engage in little manipulations of reality and our memories of that reality to suit our own needs, especially when those needs are strong. We need to learn to recognise our defences and find that having names for them will help us to notice them in ourselves and others.

Finally, the basic form of therapy has been largely set by Freud. Except for some behaviourist therapies, most therapy is still 'the talking cure', and still involves a physically and socially relaxed atmosphere. And, even if other theorists do not care for the idea of transference, the highly personal nature of the therapeutic relationship is generally accepted as important to success.

If we follow the fundamental rule of psychoanalysis and exclude as far as possible the purposive ideas of the ego, these derivatives observed in the impulses of human beings, become clearer to us. The interpretation of resistance and the id-impulse for instance demonstrates the nature of a derivative part of the ego that facilitates the finding. So, there is no interpretation merely to the unconscious components before they are represented by a preconscious derivative which the patient can recognise as such by turning attention to it. Pointing out to patient the defences used the nature of

DOI: 10.4324/9781003401322-6

defences and the possible reason for using them, how, why and against what is used, analyst guidance patient's ego to tolerate instinctual derivatives that are being made less distorted. Both in general and in treatment of refugee patient transference-resistance interpretations shows the dissociation of the ego into a part which judges reasonably and a part which experiences, the former comprehending that the latter is unseemly to the current situation but it is rather an unresolved matter from the past. These reduce anxiety and result in less distorted derivatives. These types of dissociation therefore are different from pathological dissociation and it is used as a form of self-observation with the aim of keeping certain unbearable mental contents in isolation. Working with patients with these types of defences it is important to make use of the positive transference and transient identifications.

Knowledge of the deeper psyche comes to patients through ego toleration of the unconscious. The ego participates in all analytic operations, with three main functions: (1) the execution of the id and the source of object cathexis in transference; (2) the organisation of the super-ego; (3) the institution which allows or prevents the discharge of the energy poured forth by the id.

Future-orientated intrusive thoughts

This chapter presents a general exploration of what the term 'trauma' means without a heavy psychoanalytic emphasis. Causes, consequences, dynamics and mechanisms are discussed, and particular attention is given to refugees' experience of trauma. An appreciation of what is meant by trauma is a necessary backdrop for the rest of this chapter. Stress is placed on the highly individualised nature of the experience of traumatic events; and the fact that no two people will experience a traumatic event in the same way. This is important to establish, as it is the origin and nature of individual differences in vulnerability and resilience that are investigated in this book. This provides a springboard for the discussion of post-traumatic stress as an example of vulnerability. Freud's perspectives on trauma are offered at the end, to set the psychoanalytic context of the rest of the chapter.

My findings suggest that psychoanalytic treatment provides an empirical basis for outcome-relevant treatment formulations with chronic post trauma symptoms and dissociations.

In assessment and treatment of trauma patients who present with features of unhealthy dissociations, emotional numbing and hypervigilance, depressive hopelessness, shame, fear of death and annihilation as analyst we need establish a sense of holding, containing and safety in which patient can experience his/her own body, thoughts and feelings, and able to relate to analyst as a trusted other in the process of assessments and in the group with other participants later. This interpersonal relational model permits the patient to get in touch with overwhelming impulses and self-defeating interpersonal qualities that can provide an opportunity for patient to re-construct the past, through therapeutic interactions as a containing space focuses on the primary object relational deficits.

One of the main questions in my mind from early in my career and later I look for some sort of answer in my research was: *What is it in the personality of traumatised people that makes some resilient to their traumatic experiences, but leaves others vulnerable to psychological collapse? Is it something lays in the objective external event? And what is it about the personality that enables or disables resilience?* Although my study has several limitations, such as the sample size (which was relatively small) and the setting (which was a single treatment programme), it did respond and answered what is it in the personality that makes some people to be resilient to their traumatic experiences, but leaves others vulnerable to psychological collapse. Having said this, given the potentially complex multivariate relationships among personal characteristics (e.g.: language, and other cultural factors such as ethnicity, believes, age and trauma history), I think a larger and more varied sample and a longitudinal assessment of pre and post clinical intervention and outcome is prudent and worthwhile for further explorations.

In my experience I can assert that psychoanalytically informed psychotherapy is a basis for identifying problems known and yet unknown to the patient by the patient respondents to transference interpretations. A traumatised patient's lack of response to the treatment is evidence of unhealthy dissociation and emotional impairment. Rehabilitation of chronic trauma involves a method to reverse environmental damage that is resulted in longstanding and pervasive symptomatic intensification and problems arises as the result which are likely to be exacerbated by the lack of affect regulations and impulse control of unconscious-conscious, self-organisation, and the lack essential relatedness which are associated with the early trauma in childhood. Thus, psychoanalytic treatment for traumatised patients therefore enhanced by clinician recognition of the symptomatic of PTS for which, although early childhood trauma may serve as a marker, nevertheless the trauma endured in adult life appears to best serve as a conceptual framework for clinical intervention as a start point.

Charles Darwin (1859) was in South America constructing the journey which provided many of the reflective observations that he later based The Origin of Species. When he was in Chile at the time of a large earthquake, he defined his experience as follows:

> I was on shore and lying down in the wood to rest myself. It came on suddenly and lasted two minutes (but appeared much longer). The rocking was most sensible; the undulation appeared both to me and my servant to travel from due east. There was no difficulty in standing upright but the motion made me giddy. I can compare it to skating on very thin ice or to the motion of a ship in a little cross ripple. An earthquake like this at once destroys the oldest associations; the world,

the very emblem of all that is solid, moves beneath our feet like a crust over a fluid; one second of time conveys to the mind a strange idea of insecurity, which hours of reflection would never create.

After this experience Darwin arrived at another area, in the port city of Concepción, where not a house had been left standing, and witnessed scenes of extreme despair and anguish that he found it unbearable and could not find a way to describe his feelings.

I find this historical experience is helpful when working with people who have endured trauma, especially running group with traumatised people, where the narratives are possible to become unbearable for the analyst. Analysts therefore need to be very aware of own feelings and reactions to patients' narratives in the group. We possibly will become affected by strong feelings from the patient's traumatic past that had had effects their life, which also can in the group affect the therapeutic relationship with the analyst and other participants. Hearing the stories of patients who have endured violence, persecution, imprisonments, torture or other forms of human rights violations in family, in war situations or in the community will surely have impact on both the analyst and group members on each other.

In situations that analyst feel overwhelmed by the horror narratives and emotions brought to the group, it may become difficult to remain unbiased and dispassionate to comply with the blank screen, traditionally adopted in some psychoanalytic practice. For those people who are in the process of reclaiming their lives after fleeing for their safety, blank-screen therapy will be of little help. The analyst needs to be present, and to be emotionally available to themselves and to the patient. In doing so, the analyst is committing to their own personal exploration. Providing therapeutic support to recent refugees and asylum seekers will presents challenges to our conventional training and knowledge of psychoanalysis. At the initial stages the work can be an essential debriefing, listening to patient narratives, getting familiar with characteristics of patient. This can lead to powerful feelings for the analyst who may find it tough to be a good listening-other to patient and tolerating what the patient endured, and in effect feel helpless and unable to do anything. In such circumstances, if analyst is not careful and reflective, in reality there are two patients in the room and no analyst. Often than not the analyst is the first person to hear the unrestricted version of the patient experiences, although some cultural aspects may still preventing patient to fully get engage and tell their experiences fully. Patients will surely need some time to build trust and can explore openly and associate freely to the analyst.

I learned from patients an important lessen and accept that the Western ways of accepting and discussing psychological issues may not be the same or even similar to some other cultures that many refugees are familiar. The concept of psychological pain may not be acclaimed and accepted as serious health matters and may not be accepted by many patients. Therefore, when referred the presenting problems initially is usually discussed in somatic form as the person can easily relate to the presenting and complaining of bodily pain. Thus, we need to be aware of these cultural differences in communication aspects within the therapeutic relationships. This in my experience is more challenging in the group as many cross-cultural communications may goes on at any given moment in just one session. As the analyst we need to be aware and alarmed on these for the time that the dynamic between participants may needs immediate and firm interventions to prevent negative and hostile interactions in transference between patients. With appropriate interventions we can help the group cross-cultural differences to intercultural relation and communications.

At times patients may misunderstand each other and not be aware of cultural differences which may leads them to suppress disguise some parts of their experiences. In some culture it is acceptable to talk about pain, while in other it will be considered as weakness and bad manners.

Because of the unfamiliarity of patients with each other in the group and different circumstances and backgrounds and perspectives of participants narratives, as the analyst especially at the beginning of group life we may face unpredictable challenges. It is therefore the use of supervision and consultation important source and means for us, facilitating better professional practice and enabling us to use the skills we have positively with confidence.

From the point of view of the patients in the group, I had to keep in mind for some patients who are not used to have the full attention of listening; indeed, talking in the group initially can feel unnerving, awkward or even embarrassing. By and large, after the preliminary assessment and introduction opening in the beginning of the group, people will tell their story but some participants may find it difficult in talking further. Some participants express fears, thinking the therapy service is connected to the Home Office or other officials. With such thinking, it is understandable to find it difficult to talk openly in the group. Every so often patients who engage more actively in the group are isolated, and group may be the only connections with whom they can have a meaningful conversation. As a result, the analyst also can become a significant figure in their life. People who endured abuse and are going through most frightening memory of their experiences with little or no support may use us in a variety of ways. It is our responsibility as the analyst to stay attuned with our own feelings as well as to the individual patient's needs within the group and to monitor and analyse our countertransference feelings.

Here, I am going to present a vignette about a young girl that I have worked with as an example of the group participants that I have made assessments during the process of setting up a group for young people who endured trauma. I will talk about my countertransferences towards these patients and some of my feeling that I could not analyse and make sense immediately at the time. I find it extremely challenging to manage. In my judgement, this process was one of the most challenging clinical encounters that I experienced in my career of four decades. Due to confidentiality and protections of these young people, I decided not to present the group sessions and encounters, but give example of my initial individual meetings prior to start of the group.

Tanya, who is fourteen years of age, has been coming for individual therapy for ten months with one of the child and adolescence psychotherapists. She was referred by her social worker. When I invited Tanya for assessing the possibility to invite her for the group, she was open and comfortable with talking. She was able to tell me that her father had been arrested and taken away and shortly after her mother also was arrested. She was told by her paternal aunt that her mother executed with numbers of others in her home country. She was ten at the time with a younger brother four years her junior. So, she becomes the oldest member of family and the carer for her younger sibling. Tanya herself was arrested by the military guards and like many other young girls was subjected to torture and rape, prior to coming to the UK. After her release from detention, with the help of her paternal family, she with her brother was brought to the UK.

I was not easy to listen to Tana's narratives. I felt strong empathy with this girl who was responsible for her sibling. I asked her to think if talking about her experience with others similar to her age in the group is helpful, to my surprise, she said, don't you want to know more about me before mixing me with others? I said I already discussed with her therapist's and learn much about her. She, with confidence said, there is something about you give me good feelings, i9 don't know why, but I feel connected to you different than I do with my therapist that I like very much and I am grateful to her. I said, I can hear that you would like us to meet again as you have much more to tell me. She agreed, so, I invited her to come back following week. She was much early the following week and sat in the waiting room until I called her. In this session she discloses her being witness her mother was raped and killed and said she believe somewhere out there she was watching her. I asked about her religion, she said she is not sure if she believes in God and no longer going to church. She explained she feels God is absent for her and if God exists, why does she and her family have to experience what she has? She immediately apologised to me, saying she did not want to be disrespectful and evil to me. I said, I wonder of reason that she feels she need to apologise to me by telling me her feelings and her view. In this session, while Tanya talked of her painful experiences of rape, she lifted her school uniform to show me her wound which was close to her genital and slows to heal.

Hearing Tanya's narrative and I felt I wanted to hug her and take her home with me. I remembered in our first session though she was positive about her therapist, she referred to her as being young professional, then immediately realised this is my countertransference response to her need. She needed a hug from an older person. I still felt guilty not being able to hug her, showing my affections and assuring her that everything is going to be ok. I felt there shouldn't be any different between her and other girls her age and my own daughter. I have to confess the abuse of children always will provoke a powerful feeling in me and I wish I can take them home to protect and nurture them as my own children. I had to learn over and over not to doubt that with my professional and keeping my boundaries it is possible for a child to survive such experiences as Tanya's – and I had to deal with my helplessness, and my sense of guilt and my wish to embrace her and there is no need to take them home. I had to keep hold of the knowledge that Tanya and the other girls in same or similar situations had made a skilful link and good defences to protect and rescue themselves from very young age. I had to understand that although at a comparable age I might well have been unable to cope with such atrocities as girls like Tanya, she was not me and she did cope, and I do not need to feel overwhelmed and guilty or inter-nalising her pain. In this short but challenging process, I learned that what my patient have experienced, they managed well so far – and what they needed was my help as Tanya put it 'let go of painful memories and to inte-grate in her new environment'. I had to manage my own feelings, which was not easy. Upon further thought I realised that what I was most identified with in Tanya, appeared to be her or my deep anxiety of failing to care for her younger sibling. After this insight, I felt okay to invite her to group as her narratives was not the same but similar to other young girls going to be in group. Many young people like Tanya who sought help raise questions of race, ethics, politics, economics and mental health, which may haunt the soul and remain an inescapable subject of debate.

We may take it for granted what many of the refugees and asylum seekers who arrive in the United Kingdom have experienced or witnessed devastating and debilitating violence such as war, persecution, imprisonments and torture, loss, bereavement and displacement. Although some people have experienced these atrocities externally in society, there are others who have also been abused and tortured at home by the very people who supposed to provide care to them. Some individuals may not present serious psychological symp-toms, while for many the accumulated impact of persecution, flight to a strange country, uncertainty and loss of role, status and a support network in the host country is too much to cope with. Overbearing psychological stress often presents itself in heightened incidences of anxiety, depression, panic attacks, distressing flashbacks, excessive anger or apathy, sleep disturbance, suicidal ideation, problems with memory, concentration and orientation, and psychosomatic symptoms such as headaches and back pains. The restoration of a normal life as far as possible can be the most effective way of relieving feelings of anxiety and distress, but for many refugees this is not possible and or their experiences are too overwhelming to brush aside this easily.

Within psychoanalytic perspective one of the major important is to iden-tity the early development and significant relationship. This as great part of the person character formations if remains unknown and undetected it can lead us as the analyst to misinterpret patient presenting issues. This potentially can lead to almost inescapable further psychological problems. In analytical practice it is vital that we as the analysts think in a wide range of understanding of the impact and long-term effects of the childhood trauma and distinguishes them from later trauma. We need to understand how these manifests in a range of patient's communications within the group with other participants as well as the way relating to us as the analysts as well as the narratives patients bring from other experience and interactions outside the group and clinical setting.

We know that analysts, at times perceive what patients attributing to them parallels from their own unconscious material, and respond to it with interpretation. This process for analysts as fundamental rule similar to the fundamental rule which governs the patient transference feeling, that is consists in the listening to what the patient communicates and identifying themselves with the patient's thoughts, desires, and feelings in part, while giving attention to free association; an internal communication to allow in possible thoughts and feelings to consciousness.

Here I would like to explain how I work with people vulnerabilities and my reasons for trying as much as possible focus on people strength and resiliency while working with vulnerabilities upon their experiences.

Resilience is in my view vitally important factor when we work with people who have faced a wide range of adversities with courage and grace both in personal and professional life. Many people, who have experienced significant trauma, still manage, with no or little help, to find some kind of joy and meaning in life. Among many literatures, there are two long standing psychological research of Emmy Werner (1984, 1992, 1994; Werner & Smith, 1982) and Norman Garmezy (1970, 1981, 1991, 1993; Garmezy et al., 1984) have listed some common factors typically found in resilient people. Many psychoanalysts, among them Bion (1959), Blum (1980, 1994, 2000), Cooper (1993), Ezriel (1950, 1956), Fonagy (1999), Holmes (1991), Hoggett (1992), Heimann (1950), Kernberg (1976, 1979, 1983, 1993), Hinshelwood (1994, 1997, 1999), Laplanche and Pontalis (1973), Isaacs (1952), Gordon (1995), Mace (1995), Stekel (1939), Symington (1986), have laboured to bring some air of order and systematic observation strength and vulnerability; and Stern (1985), among many others, has contributed to analytic developmental.

We know in two ways in which patients produced their memories of the past, one is by recalling and call to mind and summon up in words and one by repeating them by their behaviour generally and in the transference with the analyst and other participants in the group setting, indeed, to other relations outside the analysis in some forms. Reiteration in analytical encounter, the therapeutic relationship, the transference therefore is an expressive and informative act that is enlightening contents of the patient's unconscious. Thus transference feelings and enactments will become an important therapeutic tools and cornerstone for interpretations as principal valuable psychoanalytic technique. It could be argued that this is perhaps the most important development in the clinical practice in psychoanalytic intervention and more important than any of the multitude of developments in psychoanalytic theory, because the transference is the tool by which all the evidence and testing of the theory take place. Hinshelwood (1999) suggests:

> analysing transference is a treatment focused on the nature and extent of compliance itself. If symptoms, syndromes and diagnoses are in part (maybe a large part) socially constructed by the common attitudes amongst patients and doctors, then 'cures' are just as likely to be socially constructed from the same ingredients – social expectations and the care relationship.

Based on longstanding clinical work with people endured traumata in general and with refugees specific, I have been making a general assertion that patients more resilient to trauma exhibit, in psychotherapy, the four key characteristics that I discussed and wrote about during a few decades in detail are 'psychic space', 'sense of self', a 'listening other' and 'healthy dissociation'; these are characteristics of resiliency. Thus, although can be developed during the treatments and as the result of good therapeutic interventions whether in the group or individually, tend not to be characteristics of a vulnerable patients to begin with. To illustrate this, I will present Ana a refugee woman in her early thirties that I assessed for a group. Ana referred herself for therapy as she felt she is not able to cope anymore. In the process of assessment the evidence of resilience in her presentations was very clear and I thought she will be an excellent participant in the women group. In short period of assessments, she becomes enabled to re-connect with the original basis of her resilience which her traumatic experiences of prison and torture in her early adult life had jeopardised and almost destroyed. I recognised her characteristic way that she has managed her life after the torture was artfully alternating between relatively aggressive responses and reliably stable defences.

I will give brief historical narratives of here. Ana's parents were both in their fifties and living in her country of origin. Her father was heavily engaged in politics, which had later developed dependency on alcohol that has become a serious problem for her mother and within the wider family. Her mother was a designer. Ana described her as a woman in love with herself and distance from others. Ana was the youngest of two, with brother senior to her who was loving and protective towards her. She had a normal birth and according to her parents she had been a happy and healthy child and developed well. She told me that her difficulties began in her adolescence, when her father began drinking out of control and his behaviour become somehow irrational. She expressed that her father always was loving and caring to her, but his new being under influence of alcohol creates great fears in her and she start feeling guilty and also unwanted. She felt that her mother was engaged with her own world in fashion and her friend. Her mother was not present to help her during those important periods, her brother was also left home for university and she was feeling that she left totally insecure, vulnerable and unshielded. She felt that she needed strong connections and she was searching to find a closed friendship within her peer group at school. She soon discovered many of her friends experiencing drug and alcohol that she hated. This stressed her immensely, so, she decided that she has to cut her tie to those friends and turned to books and reading about history and politics and soon become involved in an opposition political activity.

At the time we met, Ana was new in the UK and had just started to improve her English and said she feels dead if she cannot work. She was separated from her partner and living part of the week with her son, and was on good terms with her ex-partner, sharing with him the responsibility for the son. She shared the same political view with father of her son and they both have had same experiences of persecution, imprisonments and torture and because of their son, they together have decided to leave their home country and seek refuge, before being arrested again and may be executed. After her arrival in the UK, she felt at loss, hence she thought of seeking help to be able to find a way forward and stand on her own feet as she put it. She said she is getting some help from state and hate to continue this for a long time. Interestingly enough, she said some people call it government benefit that is not correct. This is hard working people money we are giver, it is amazing and helpful to have it, but always have to be for short period and not long term, unless someone have disability and not able to do any work. She disclosed to me with clear awareness that she knows she is suffering with depressions, but she does not want to take medications that her GP suggest. She said she really want to do anything in her power not allow her psychological problems affect her son. I asked her what does she think is making her depress now. She said, she knows that leaving her country she would be losing her social world. She loved her family, her many good and trusting friends, her home, her work and many other things, but she would risk her life if she would stay and she could not do that to her son and other loving people in her life, she said. She explained how sometimes she find the life to be too challenging here, but she knows this is temporary and she has to pass this and learn to live in her new environment with hope she can go back when situations in her country changed.

In total, for assessment, I met Ana for six sessions, to ensure group will be appropriate, and then I proposed to her that I would like her to join the group. Surprisingly, she welcomed this and agreed. She said she needed help to find ways for her to see the present in terms of her past; and she is sure she can learn from other women in the group. She then asked me if in a particular period she find it difficult can I see her again individually. I said any participants in the group who may need extra support beyond group, I will gladly allocate a therapist for her, but I will not see group members outside the group. She laughed and said I like it; you don't want to behave like my mother who always favoured my brother. I was impressed and thought this woman has amazing insight. During our work together, I had to learn a great deal about how to monitor Ana's conscious and unconscious processes. At times, she could become very defensive and there were occasions when I could feel at loss with her. I had to be very careful to monitor my countertransference and my unconscious for not allow my issues becoming disruptive in our therapeutic encounters. I was very aware from the outset that in my countertransference, I liked Ana and her attitude to life very much and I was constantly enchanted by her and thought she was delightful to work with. And of course, she was as I suspected a great participant to help other women in the group. Although she was able to talk about her depression and anxiety, she also showed considerable resilience. I thought her depression and anxiety is not at the alarming stage and it is normal reactions to her abnormal situations. In the process of our individual meetings, I could identify in her a happy little girl whose life was disrupted and who had not had an opportunity yet to work through the trauma she had endured by political oppression, consequent persecution and torture. I had the impression that she relied on her main defences as high achiever and a good lever of communications with powerful vocabulary is a pattern denoted and be a sign of her early life to impress her mother and to compete with her beloved brother. She presented defences, which I considered relatively healthy, such as humour, repression, displacement, suppression, and intellectualisation, indeed healthy dissociations to control her feelings and affect that surfaced. In the group Ana continued with the same patterns of behaviour and relating to prevent a breakdown, while also was mindful to other group members and she would on right timing would change the subject of her discussion or discloser not to make overwhelming feelings in the group. In one of the session when one of member for first time was talking about her last communications with her husband before him being executed, Ana very naturally said today I have nothing to contribute and allocate her time to that member. This was touching for others in the group and set a level of care between woman afterward and this become habitual for all in the group.

In the transference, the relationship patients established with me in the group, like any other object-relationship, was made up of a never-ending complementary movement of introjection and projection, envy, jealousy, sibling rivalry and competitiveness. Where the introjected object tended to occupy too much space in the group interactions, I considered that participants' capacity is to project that part of themselves onto me or each other would help to differentiate and separate the self of that person from the object consciousness. On occasions when the group members felt connected and emotionally settled, then, the separation-anxiety becomes excessive, and projective identification tends to increase, so that the interpretation of projections, to the extent that it could create insight in participant's mind, contributes to abandoning narcissistic identification. Projective identification then encouraged the formation of stronger ego structures, by gathering concurrently the essential aspects of the ego, with the continuous reorganisation, representing some improvement of the ego, in constant search for realisation and unification. This process was complicated and challenging, but when I could manage to contain it and facilitate the group, and, when happens, it will bring great insights to all members. I call it moments of meetings the human genuine contacts.

Sometimes when a trauma is too horrendous, an individual psyche responds by simply denying the existence of the traumatic experience. Mind and body act together to expel painful experiences, especially when the person feels vulnerable and does not see a way out. Pain, therefore, becomes an alien substance like an antigen, stimulating repression as a reaction that will counteract the pain without the relief – much as an antibody would. Although the repression of trauma keeps participants in the group from feeling overwhelmed, it also keeps the person safe. The immune reaction of repressing pain creates a state of neutrality, a sense of existing behind a wall where life seems to be going on beyond one's reach – somewhere out there. The recovery of wellbeing, in such instances, depends on gaining or regaining resilience. By doing that, the individual in the group and empathy members towards each other will increase psychic space for further exploration and reflection towards a better sense of self and others.

In my view dissociation and resilience are important for the initial and ongoing assessments of patients' psychological wellbeing or lack of it. This is not replacement or substitute to other important psychoanalytic theory and concepts and their clinical implications but, in my view the relationship of resilience quality and people personality and coping styles has been undermined or unattended.

I will present an example here. I shall be keeping respects for confidentiality of the discussions and interactions in the group. I first will discuss some significant perspectives on the qualitative research with psychoanalytic practice. Then I present a qualitative process analysis of a young patient I call Ivan, who I after a process of assessments invited to join the young man group where his language was used in the group. Ivan had suffered intense life-threatening trauma. In the beginning he was not able to articulate his experiences. Having said this, he has changed in the process and was able to connect in the group and express his feeling especially when other group members talked about their experience of trauma. I will be giving a case history as an example of data for analysis and will discuss the methods used as an example of the way in which I worked with Ivan and other young patients that I was assessing for the group. I set my first task to listen, collect and organise the experiences and with each patient to make meanings. With this particular group and the culture they come from, I was aware presenting or talking about vulnerability was not possible in the beginning for them. In order to create a safe and containing environment, I needed to do more than just making meanings with most of the patients, including Ivan. I used a narrative construction based on certain assumptions. Although Ivan has self-narrative, it was concealed or he would retreat from it. Sometimes he would present another narrative of the third person which he does not directly related to him and he did not need to relate to it as his own. So, I work on the basis that the aim of our therapeutic encounter is to start working with him this way. So, with a gentle interpretations I introduce the idea that Ivan wish to talk on the non-self-narrative which exists in him, but for now his own real narrative is out of our reach as he wishes to retreating from it. I told him I respect his wishes and invite him to join the group. I explained, it will be beneficial for him to join the group that other participants have same or similar experiences. With hesitations, he agreed. This of course is not ordinary discipline and one cannot say how we can establish and know for sure if it is patients' subjectivity and or my own. And how could I know that the hidden narrative of Ivan is really there in him and it is not my expectations which he feels obliged to respond. All these reservations and doubts are admissible, but we only can work with our knowledge and hypotheses.

In the process of setting up this group and assessing the young patients optimistically, I needed to revisit some of the classic literature, and I have found numerous Freud works that predominantly concentrate on the elaboration of psychoanalytical technique and religious and cultural history helpful in regards to reconstructions. These including *Totem and Taboo* (Freud, 1913g), *The Theme of the Three Caskets* (Freud, 1913h) and *The Claims of Psychoanalysis to Scientific Interest* (Freud, 1913e), his metapsychological works *Instincts and Their Vicissitudes* (Freud, 1915d) and *Repression and The Unconscious* (Freud, 1915g), and his essay *Thoughts for the Times on War and Death* (Freud, 1915b) that he elaborates his ideas about the outbreak of the First World War and the consequences of the conflict between culture and instinctual life.

I have furthermore revisited Ezriel's (1956) proposition on the methodology of psychoanalysis that he had discussed that we need to clarify the discipline of psychoanalysis in our research for out outcome to be regarded scientifically validated. He made points with emphasis how the conventional method of investigation in observation of events in the 'here and now', as opposed to history or archaeology which reconstructed particular events from the past in order to explain present conditions and that psychoanalysis is widely assumed to fall within the latter category. Freud compared the analyst to the archaeologist in the way he 'digs up' a patient's past in the form of memories, associations and so on. Ezriel (1956) suggested that this view missed the very 'here and now' aspect of material which was 'unconsciously selected for (the analyst) by the subject of his investigation, the patient ... presented to him ... both spontaneously and in response to the analyst's interventions' (p. 31). In attempting to understand a patient's behaviour, he asked himself what made the patient do and say particular things in front of him at specific moments in time. Then he passed interpretative comments back to the patient, who he said was 'a kind of reality testing and arguably the essence of psychoanalytic therapy' (ibid., p. 39). He demonstrates how the use of recordings and the playing back of sessions made it possible to test hypotheses of human behaviour through closely observing interactions between the patient and analyst. He also noted the importance of transference in the therapeutic process, suggesting that it could have both positive and negative effects on the patient and result in either improvement or deterioration in its 'aim at avoiding frightening impulses towards the analyst' (ibid., p. 47).

The additional specific concept that I have taken into account as a relevant concept in working with group of patients experienced human right violations is John Steiner's (1993) 'psychic retreats' that is states of mind into which patients can withdraw in order to avoid or escape anxiety, mental pain, indeed psychotic breakdown. In such state of mind, patients become restricted in their lives and can feel 'stuck' in their treatment, or experience a total withdrawal from reality. The embodiment of Steiner (1993) discussion that is very helpful, relational. Important dynamics I have learned from Steiner as an analyst if I am able to successfully contain those elements projected onto me by the patient, and not turn to critical or hostile interpretations then I help the patient to feel understood. This relational interaction is the processes which lead to improvement, greater integration and development in patient and creates positive change in the group and participants interactions with each other and with me. This is specifically useful in working with people whose lives have been disturb by trauma and whose experiences have made them lonely, isolated, out of touch with others, and in some cases out of real touch with their own self. This is quite important as in the psychoanalytic literature our traumatic experience start at birth and not the external trauma experienced in adult life. Though patient childhood trauma is impotent in development and personality formation, a refugee patient may present extra and specific schemata that can be the result of external trauma in their life.

In our clinical practice as the goal and objective of our practice is a therapeutic dialogue, there will be a journey from the reality of the speaking, that is, patient presentation and analyst understanding by means of interpretation. The process and reflection of the therapeutic process and our assessments of outcome usually are through visiting our notes, transcripts of analysis and working through, as well as verbal discussions in supervision or consultation. The point of this process is not to ground the text or the result as part of the validation process, but to impart fact or knowledge. Consequently, the emphasis can be on pragmatic validation, that is, the advantageousness and helpfulness of the results in patients' life. The beauty advantage of psychoanalytic therapeutic process is based on an open feed-back system, where both patient and analyst are constantly making more or less explicit adjustments to and with the other. As a result, the emphasis on the tentativeness of the conclusion in reality within relationship dyad can only be in qualitative methods. The intention of the psychoanalytical ther-apeutic intervention in the process is to broaden and expand the patients' knowledge about themselves and their relation to others, and this is achiev-able within the group dynamics with other group participants and with the analyst, and without doubt become character building tools with other rela-tions outside therapy. The use of language by interpretations made will broadening participant's prospects. The narratives therefore will be under-stood in context; indeed the first interpretation to the context may not always the final in a particular tome in particular sessions, but also can be the beginning of a journey towards an insight to be gain in a process.

In my view psychoanalytic approach is the most useful in treating people. Psychoanalytic validation is by the qualitative methods that are presented as text, narratives, dialogues and descriptions and cannot be reduced to quan-titative measurement of fixed categories and ticking boxes. The reduction of an often-unmanageable quantity is determined not only by statistical princi-ples, but, amongst other things, by the point of view that is consciously chosen. This includes observation, the attribution of meaning or significance to historical facts, and the researcher's choice of material to be analysed for presentation. In qualitative method the criteria for election and the way of evaluating outcome are based on phenomena significant from the therapeutic point of view, not on their statistical mean. The process aims at and focuses on the new and specific phenomena that are analysed and in their context. Psychoanalytic evaluations are by text creates the structure of meanings, through written case vignettes, conveyed to the reader. This is an example of good human psyche study. It makes a distinction between the use of the word and the significant meaning and its effect on the text, based on individual patient presentation – and aims to relate to one's internal structure and the way it is constructed – that is – the internal coherence and rationality for validity, or the lack of it that corresponds to the shared meaning or under-standing, constructing a scheme for knowledge and theories for interpreta-tion within psychoanalysis. The significance of a text therefore must be understood as something about the world and/or as having a message about a particular as phenomenon which may not be shared between patients and analyst, at least at the beginning. This is in contrast with the aim of quanti-tative methods that design with the intention to determine whether or not a speculative property is presented as a mean.

It is important to note that as part of our training in psychoanalysis we learned to observe in session presentations on a scale of seconds and minutes (working with individual patient) and to ensure to have ongoing careful monitoring and evaluation; and to evaluate the outcome changes in people's regular weekly supervision on each individual patient as part of our clinical training. Apart from process record for supervision, write the progress reports once every six months for each trainee patient. This is done by considering aspects of what are identified as the person's problematic experiences and how they are negotiated, by studying each one separately and over time. The trainee analyst needs to consider how the patient's experiences are understood as derivatives of distressing and troublesome experiences; how they may be understood within psychoanalytic perspective, able to observe and analyse dialogical patterns as they appear in relational scenarios, taking into consideration complex psychological schemata through being with others, the transference, expressed emotion in explicit and implicit pattern behaviour; and the pattern of conveying significance meaning.

All this are a learning process that will help the analyst observe and examine patient's presentation of unwanted thoughts and ambiguous or unstructured feelings. With interpretation, clarification the analyst's job is to explain, elucidate, identify and distinguish the problem, and to help the patient further explorations to verbalise thoughts and increase insight. This is done in an atmosphere created for working through, enhancing and developing the patient's ability for problem-solving, creating ego strength, autonomy, resilience and mastery. A patient may enter therapy with problems at any level of assimilation. In the process, continuum movement of any gap identified can be considered progress on an individual basis. If, in the initial meetings, analyst can become aware of some aspects of resilience in a patient, that will provide a basis groundwork to use and build on that part of personality; and also provide possibilities for patient to exercise their ability to deal with vulnerabilities in the process. This is a dialogical view on psychoanalytic that is coherent with object relation, focuses on encounters between the patient and the analyst's inner world, both at the conscious and unconscious level. Thus, all of speech, including the inner speech of the patient is addressing the listener – that is the analyst – which is consciously or unconsciously becomes part of the process as a second party by transference. This of course may be presented in the form of third party at conscious level of the patient – that is to say, there is always something beyond the immediate transference object. The dual disposition of responsive understandings allows the message to live in the analyst without being given a final meaning, but can allow a new meaning to appear. This is the integral and essence of holding and containing of analyst like a mother and baby.

Another importance factor in qualitative methods in psychoanalytic research and evaluation is the element that analysts will take into consideration when a patient talks about an experience. Thus, like a mother and baby making the transition from the non-symbolised position; where experience is represented mostly as bodily signs and behaviour – to an embryonic and basic ability to formulate traces of the experience and verbalise it. When dialogue is about the experience, the patient establishes the ability to place it in a particular time perspectives, then can place it in relation to atypical social and psychological contexts. The analyst does and needs to carefully observe words, sounds and expressions, making distinctions between when the patient is speaking about their experience – that is speaking about a particular experience and reflecting on the experience. In the later, when patient reflecting on the experience, the patient and analyst are able to explore the emotional meaning of experience together, and in the group this may be richer with other group members participating insightfully. This will provide patient prospect to look at the reorganisation of the self and therefore to open up a readiness for sublimation, integration and further resiliency. At each level the analyst as a listener is situated in specific transference positions by the patient who consciously or unconsciously needs or demands a specific form of responsive understanding. For that reason, the analyst's ability and willingness to learn to make these distinctions is necessary in forming knowledge of the way the word is organised, articulated and communicated by the patient, along the expressions presented. Patterns and sequences may frequently be derived from the patient's self-narrative that imply how the person relates to various aspects of themselves. Communication patterns mediated by non-verbal signs and metaphorical aspect of meanings in the patient-analyst discourse correspondingly need to be identified in transference. The analyst's countertransference feelings and fantasies are other sources for identifying non-verbal communication patterns. To summarise in order to observe and analyse each situation a number of steps need to be taken in the process. Firstly, to define the patient's position in terms of mutually explicit and implicit object positions in which the meaning and presentation are observed, identified and by interpretations clarified. The self-aspect presentation of 'I' or 'Me' and 'You' in patient presentations to be understood and clarified. The analyst needs to learn from what position the patient is speaking and to differentiate that is, which 'I' or 'Me' is speaking to which 'You' – as all refer to different parts of the self – and in which, patient can associates with easily, and or the part which may be difficult for patient to make direct associations. The ways in which a patient can or will relate to their wishes, fantasies and fears, and how these are presented, along with what is being addressed. Further, it is the analyst's job to follow the development of these perceptions throughout the identified the sequences and seeking clarifications. To specify the 'I' and the 'You' positions as material in the process and further clarify when more than one position is presented in one relations and reasoning for it. This is specifically very important when working with refugees and other traumatised people who have been affected by multiple traumas, and may have difficulties to express themselves partly due to language and cultural barriers and partly fear of being themselves in the present of others. It is imperative for the analyst to clarify and understand before offering interpretation for working through, ensuring what has been presented by patients.

Here I will bring another brief Vignette to demonstrate data collection in psychanalysis. Mahmood was a young refugee who had been imprisoned for two years, severely tortured and forced to witness other people being tortured, including his wife, his sister and his child. He, after discharge from prison left his country to escape from further persecutions and lost contact with his entire family. Later he tried to trace his family members through Red Cross in the UK, without any success. In the referral letter it was indicated that he was making frequent visits to his GP, almost on a daily basis unless he has other appointments, with psychosomatic presentations and was advised to think about whether his problems might be psychological. After consideration he informed his GP that he is keen to receive psychological help. Mahmood and I had three sessions for assessment to decide whether I could be helpful to him. He presented himself as somebody who could avoid and resist accepting he wanted a quick fix. In response to my question about why he sought help, he conveyed that it was because his GP impressed on him. I said it seems that he was not here because he think it may be helpful to him to deal with the traumatic experiences inflicted on him and the loses he endured, but because he needed other people's approval that he is listening to them, in this case is his GP and his case worker in Red Cross and I wonder if he found himself constantly worried to disappoint others in their view of him. Looking down at his knees, becoming quite tearful but controlling himself he shook his head. He then start recalling occasions where he had in fact explained to others that he was vulnerable and in need of help, hence, instead of being helped, only to receive a response of dislike and rejection, which he found himself ended up with disappointment and further pain and stress. It became apparent that his avoidance was perhaps a sign and an effort to cover up and cope with rejection and helplessness. I said, thank you for sharing your experiences and how you asking for help has been disappointing experience for you. I then asked I wonder if this narrative was his response to my question about my understanding of his current state of mind and seeking help. He became thoughtful in silence. In this particular moments Mahmood talking about the importance of not disclosing too much of his problems for fear of making other people worry and not just experiencing rejection. This way, although he could be aware of his difficulties, he did not want with his action cause himself further pain on rejection or being misunderstood. In response to my enquiries for clarification Mahmood was insistent that I needed to understand his position and not see it in terms of him being a defensive patient without good reasons. He said:

> When a person from my country comes to see me, I cannot start talking negative to disappoint the person with my problem or what happened to me ... therefore I try not to talk about my problem, you know, you have to protect yourself and others from further pain.

I thought it is important to present a brief vignette of Mahmood here and his ways of relating to himself with 'I', 'Me' and 'You'.

I formulate Mahmood's presentation of his experiences that his thoughts and memories of the atrocities he had endured and offered interpretations that he would feel needy and helpless and receives rejection and humiliation, which in turn made him angry and frustrated and do not want to be open with others. Such feeling also activated another state of mind where he experienced murderous way of thinking and hatred towards others he interacted and deemed to be helpless with. He was responsive to these interpretations by saying, 'I never thought about it this way and until now actually I didn't know I am angry with them'.

My objective and hope in session of assessment process with Mahmood was to first gain a thorough history and become familiar with the material he was presenting. These were doing by listening to him and facilitate possibility of thinking and reflecting. The group therapy would be long-term and by gaining ability to listen to others in the group without pre-judgments of not being liked potentially he could recover from those negative thinking. So, my job during the assessments was to encourage him to listen to what is presented here carefully. If, he is in doubt, ask without fear to be provided with explanations and further give attention to the verbal and non-verbal aspects of the interactions with others. I had to be careful in communicating with him at this stage and that paid off well. Mahmood's behaviour changed. In one of the last session before the group, in the beginning he said: 'I feel you are not your usual self.' And that was correct, so I was pleased to see he is becoming able to relate. At that point, I knew I can invite him to be one of the participants in the group. The structure of how analysed Mahmood and worked with him to dealt with or coped with his experience was central to the process assessment to enable him to join a group without fear of being rejected or hated by others. By doing so, I then, identified his strength as well as his weakness and aspects of what may be called mental health strategy as the foundation to overcoming the effects of trauma for his autonomy and resiliency.

Chapter 6

Important psychoanalytical concepts in work with people who have endured trauma

Freud's *Mourning and Melancholia* outlined the major tenets of a revised model of the mind that Freud termed object relations (Freud, 1914, 1917c, 1923, 1926a), and following this Klein (1946) and other contemporary psychoanalysts further developed the object relation theories that are important in working in the group, indeed with people affected by trauma. The object relations theory is important in general in psychoanalysis and much relevant in working with refugees. By taking into consideration both internal and external reality and intra-psychic relationships, the perception of self and its relation to the external world, and a distinction between secure and insecure connections patients may have both in early development or in later life. In this chapter I highlight what sort of psychoanalytical ideas in practice I find to be important to focus when working with refugees. The drive theory and its development, the object relation theory, the concept of the self I leaned to constitute important factors in my work with refugees both with individual and in the group. Ability or inability for mourning is also important for people experienced many losses, including refugees.

Key helpful ideas in psychoanalysis

I start with the principle of Freud's (1915b) pioneering theory of the unconscious as a broad spectrum of human behaviour that can be explainable in terms of the hidden mental states and processes. This is one of the main differences between psychoanalysis and other forms of therapy. Psychoanalysis doesn't consider the neurotic behaviours as causally enigmatic perplexing behaviour that can disappear with approach insists on being treatable. Instead psychoanalysis considers and deals with it as behaviour for which it is meaningful to seek an explanation, by searching for causes in the mental states of the individual patients, with observing dreams, slips of the tongue and obsessive behaviour that are determined by hidden causes in the person's unconscious mind, and can reveal in covert form what would otherwise is unknown. The cause of neurotic or even psychotic behaviour is not in the conscious mind.

DOI: 10.4324/9781003401322-7

The implication of unconscious mental states is that the mind is not able to identify and therefore not able to make change with consciousness, although it can be an object of consciousness laying below the surface, exerting a dynamic that can determine influence upon the part which is compliant to direct assessment of the conscious mind. Greatly associated with this are instincts as the principal motivating forces in the mental space that motivate and invigorate the mind in its functions. Eros is life instinct covers the self-preserving and erotic instincts, and, Thanatos is death instinct which covers the instincts towards aggression, self-destruction, and harshness. The critics of psychoanalysis limit Freud's theory with their assumption that all human behaviours spring from motivations which are sexual in their origin, but motivations derive from Thanatos are not sexually motivated, it is urge to destroy the source of all sexual energy in the annihilation of the self. Freud (1905b) indeed gave sexual drives as important and central in human behaviour, arguing that sexual drives exist and can be discerned in children from birth, and sexual energy or libido is motivation force in adult life. However, the term sexuality covers any form of pleasure which is derived from bodily sensation. Thus his theory of instincts or drives is principally that the human being is energised or driven from birth by the desire to develop, assimilate and enhance pleasure from bodily touch and contact. These hidden aspects of the psyche may affect traumatised person ability to live a fulfilling life after a traumatic event.

Freud's (1905b) theory of infantile sexuality is an integral part of a developmental theory which considers that traumatic childhood events can leave negative effects upon the adult individual, and that early childhood sexual experiences are factors in the fortitude strength of personality in adult life. Instincts or drive theory indicates that from birth we are driven in our actions by the desire for pleasure, to gain release as following:

- The *oral stage* of development –the act of sucking.
- The *anal stage* –the stage in which the locus of pleasure and energy release is the anus, particularly in the act of defecation.
- The *phallic stage* –development and interest in sexual organs as a place of pleasure.
- The *Oedipus complex* or *Electra complex* – that is the development of a deep sexual attraction for the parent of the opposite sex, and a hatred of the same sex parent.

Gives rise to socially derived feelings of guilt, as we recognise that we can never displace our powerful parent. In a male, it puts the child at risk which he perceives when he pursues the sexual attraction for his mother, he fears to be harmed by his father. This is the castration anxiety. As male attraction for mother and hatred for the father is not acceptable it should be repressed, the child may resolves the conflict of the Oedipus complex by coming to identify with the parent of the same sex. This is in the latency period, in which sexual motivations become much less pronounced and will lasts until puberty when mature genital development begins and the pleasure drive focuses around the genital area.

In the developmental stages a movement through a series of conflicts is necessary and the positive efficacious resolutions of these processes are essential for psychological health. Many psychological weaknesses and complaints, particularly hysteria can easily be traced back to disturbances in these stages and unresolved conflicts which interrupt the usual pattern of development.

The id, ego, and super-ego

It can be said that Freud's (1915b) account of the unconscious and the structure of mind is similar to Plato's account of the nature of psychological well-being, which Freud formulated with the establishment of a harmonious relationship between the three structural elements which distinguish and constitute the mind to id, ego and superego.

- The *id* is the unconscious mind, the part of the mind in which the instinctual sexual drives for pleasure are situated.
- The *ego* is the conscious self of dynamic tensions and interactions between the id and the superego which has the task of integrating conflicting demands with the requirements of external reality. All objects of consciousness reside in the ego.
- The *superego* comprises of socially acceptable behaviour and morals that are learned mainly from the parents and have been internalised. The superego is an unconscious screening mechanism seeking to control the pleasure-seeking drives of the id with the imposition of restrictive directions.

Common defences

Defences are group of operations aimed at the reduction of change likely to threaten our strength, integrity and constancy. The ego is constituted as an agency which embodies this stability and strives to maintain it. In practice, its action is extended to representations of symbols, memories and phantasies of situations that are incompatible with the individual's balance and therefore is not pleasurable for the ego function. There are a number of defences more relevant than others in the context of patients intrapsychic. Our mind possesses a variety of defences to prevent conflicts from becoming too acute, including:

- repression;
- fixation;
- denial;

- disavowal;
- displacement;
- projection (in the form of altruistic surrender and reaction formation);
- introjections and identification (specifically identification with aggressor);
- intellectualisation and rationalisation; and
- sublimation.

Repression

Repression is one of our defences which involves a movement back and forth in psychological time when we face with stress, especially when we are troubled or frightened, we can see that our behaviour may become primitive. For example, a refugee yet uncertain of the good will of the analyst may present for some time as silly and thoughtless and trivial. This is not uncommon and adopted by many refugee patients in the hope of surviving the trauma by not remembering the events. This I find to be quite important with person experiences torture and sexual or physical violent and humiliations. In such situations instinctual impulses behave in a manner which the superego deems to be reprehensible; consequently, the mind pushes it away, repressing it into the unconscious. This is the central defence mechanism by which the ego seeks to avoid internal conflict and pain, and to reconcile reality with the demands of both id and superego. The repressed instinctual drive but cannot be destroyed and will continue to exist in the unconscious from where it exerts a determining force upon the conscious mind, and can give rise to the dysfunctional behaviour characteristic of neuroses. Dreams and slips of the tongue can uncover what is happening in the unconscious, and this is why they are significant and interpretation represents key part of psychoanalytic therapy.

Repression is central and of the essence in working with refugee patients, as many have to repress both internal and external trauma. This is vitally important in group dynamics as there are almost at all times there is possibility that the person project their internal conflicts to the external person with hope to deal with their own reality. This process may bring the danger of feeling comfortable by colluding with another participant in the group who may like to collude with the victim role and not taking responsibility for one own life issues and experience after the trauma. One of the tasks of the analyst in such occurrences working with such group therefore is to find what types of repressions are causing the neurotic symptoms or even stronger acting out, by delving into the unconscious mind of the patient to bring the repressions to consciousness and allowing the ego to confront them. It is important to bear in mind at all times the patient's external reality and its real effects on internal being. We need to distinguish which problems stem from within the patient's psyche and which stem from without as the result of particular group dynamics.

Fixation

Fixation is the state of mind when person may be obsessed with an attachment to another human, animal or dead object. This is the result of disturbances during one of the developmental stages. For example for a person who has not been receiving appropriate gratification during one or more developmental stage, the conflict is, at least in part, developmental; if so, which specific stage has left strong impression which can confirm earlier personality formation prior to adult trauma which may have been pathology that reflect throughout person adult life.

Denial

Denial is another main defence mechanisms associated closely with working with some refugees. Denial involves blocking external events from awareness, when a situation is too overwhelming to handle. Denial is a form of self-deception that protects the individual from fears and threats to the self and involves exaggerated perceptions of control. Denial can also have positive aspects that protect the integrity of the self-concept by distorting reality in a self-enhancing way during the crisis. It promotes a sense of mastery and control that leads to lower levels of anxiety.

Disavowal

Freud (1914a) put forward the concept of disavowal, describing the simultaneous acknowledgement of and blindness to the traumatic event. Disavowal is a distinct form of denial involving self-deception in the face of accurate perception, and is often recurrently used to deal with stressful situations of the traumatic events as and when happening and the memory of experience is later.

Displacement

Displacement is one of the tormenting defence mechanisms frequently unspoken but observed to take on by some people endured traumas including refugees. It is the redirection of an impulse onto a substitute being directed at recipient object. For example, if a person has a strong desire, but that desire is too threatening, the desires displaced onto someone or something that can serve as emblematic substitute. A special form of displacement is the act of turning against the self, where the person becomes their own substitute target. Displacements is typically used to defend against negative impulses like hatred, anger, and aggression.

Projection

Projection is almost the opposite of displacement or turning against the self. It involves the tendency to see our own unacceptable desires in other. For example, with some patients who are coming from culture that homo-sexuality is not accepted or in some country will be persecuted and punished, I observed some people who have homosexual feelings and interest but not able to acknowledge or peruse the feelings may present themselves as an angry homophobic and turn into more and more disturbed and complain about the presence of homosexuality in Western society. I usually find this type of presenting matters helpful for patients and find it helpful as the analysts to move directly to the presenting matter. This is altruistic surrender, one form of projection that initially appears as the opposite of submission. I present it here as an important psychoanalytical theory for analysing when we are faced with situation patients attempt to fulfil own needs through others. In the extreme form of projections, there is always danger that one living life entirely for and through others. For example a political activist who has been raped in prison may disassociate with the personal experience of being rapped as the weapon of torture and as a substitute and replacing own trauma become an active campaigner against rape. A similar defence to this is reaction formation, that involves transforming an unacceptable impulse into its opposite to be acceptable. For example a depressed mother who is not able to cope with her responsibility and is angry with her child may become overly anxious with her child and showing excessive concerns and overly affectionate.

Introjection

Introjection involves taking someone else's disposition characteristics as one's own, to solve various emotional problem and complexity. Introjection is sometimes called identification. Identification with the aggressor is a common reaction with people who have been abused and tortured. It is a version of introjection that focuses on the adoption of negative or feared traits. For example for a person who is frightened of the perpetrator can subjugate that fear by becoming more like them. This is identification with the aggressor, an intrapsychic conflict that can contain aspects of the external world which created after the external trauma. Such conflicts are between divergent of self-representations, both accepted part and a rejected part of the self-representing identification with a degraded object. There are conflicts between strong or weak, dominant or submissive, sadistic or masochistic. Such defences are the internalised reproductions and repetitions of the interpersonal dynamics of abuse, an expression of split part of the self, identified with the aggressor. A famous example of identification with the aggressor is the 'Stockholm Syndrome' where the hostages were positively sympathetic towards their abductors. Another example is prisoners' experi-ences with the Nazi prison officers studied by Jacobsen (1959) who held themselves behaving like their guards, as they go through anxious depersonalisation catastrophes.

Intellectualisation

Intellectualisation is usually presented on a rather somewhat conscious level. It is a cognitive alteration of the facts to make an event or impulse less intimidating. We may habitually perform in our behaviour and discussion when on some occasions we stipulate justification for ourselves. For a well defended person with perceptive ego, this defence comes so easily that they may not always be actually aware when they are doing it. Rationalisation similarly is the cognitive distortion of the facts to make an event or an impulse less intimidating or frightening. We do it often enough on a fairly conscious level when we provide ourselves with justify motive and reason.

Sublimation

Sublimation is the transformation of unacceptable impulse, whether it is sexual desire, anger or fear, into a socially acceptable and valuable appearance which can be used positively. For example, someone with strong anger and hostility may become a hunter, a butcher, a surgeon or an athlete. Someone suffering from a great deal of social anxiety may become an organiser, or a researcher. Many refugees may in the new country and new environment find different prospects, learning to embrace and assimilate to the new culture in the host country and sublimate to a new way of life.

Most of defences can be in the form of denial and disavowals, even if we are not conscious of making them. Whether we are conscious of using them or not, all defences serve to hide the truth and take us away from our real selves and preventing us from our reality. A useful way of understanding the mechanism of defences when working with refugees particularly in the group setting is to see them as a combination of denial and disavowal, displacement, repression, introjection, projection, projective identification, with various kinds of intellectualisation and rationalisations. These are used as protective factors to survive the atrocities that many refugees have tolerated and lived on. The challenge and dilemma I observed in the group settings was the facts that in many group encounter the protective effect of such defences, if I wanted to deal with particular defences with direct interpretations, I could restricted the group and may isolate a participant unable to cope. This potentially could create unmanageable negative transference within the group causing all denied and stored anxieties to come rushing forward and hypothetically cause collapse of analysis in the group.

Fetishism

Fetishism or perversions represent other defence strategies for not dealing with trauma, which I observed used often by refugee patient in response to losses and their impact. The construction and deployment fetishism and perversions intended to eliminate the traces of the trauma and loss. Some patient behaviour could result in the use of perverse and or fetish that may be contrasted with different mode or symbolic behaviour. This could be the inability or refusal to mourn traumatic events and is a strategy for undoing the need for mourning by means of phantasy, simulating a provision of intactness, placing the origin of loss elsewhere. These types of defence usually turns either to aggression or to fetishism which may discharge one from the problem of having to reconstitute and reconstruct one's self-identity under posttraumatic syndromes. It is not difficult to recognised in this function of a person presentations the effects of trauma is for the foreseeable time have been on hold and ongoing. Through disavowal of the other's castration, thus of the consciousness of an external reality, a person can partially at the cost of a psychic splitting, maintain its certainty in the existence of symbol. Along these lines, the splitting typically makes the object of an exaggerated and perverse conflict in the fear of castration. Perjure oneself between isolation, cancellation, and denial, which Freud (1926b) defined as psychic mechanism, that will allow the unconscious to penetrate the conscious mind without there being any acceptance of the elimination. The concept of the splitting of the ego is Freud's (1936) deliberations linking to fetishism. He suggested that 'the fetish is a substitute for the woman's penis that the little boy once believed in and … does not want to give up'. Fetishism is made possible by a very specific form of denial, one that Freud called 'Verleugnung', a term that has been rendered in the Standard Edition as 'disavowal' (ibid., pp. 152–153).

Dissociation

Dissociation is a response to trauma used by some people. I consider some types of dissociations a healthy defence as a successful act of leaving the organisation of one's world relatively intact and preventing a total psychological collapse. People, who are unable to accomplish this successfully, can encounter fragmentation of the self and of the perception of the world. Psychoanalytic interventions conjure up to ego strength as a necessity for the existence of strength and resilience in the mind of the individual. In the group encounter different individual minds may respond differently to the same objective occurrences. The notion of dissociation is useful for explorations independent and group interactions in search for alternative for participants to understand individual differences in any given moments in the group. Grotstein (1978) developed a concept of inner space as the capacity to experience space as a principal mechanism of ego autonomy, which seems to have arisen from the immature sensations upon the foetal skin at birth, in so doing 'awakening the skin with its sense receptors into its functions as a surface, as a boundary between self and non-self, and as a container of self' (p. 56). With regard to the development of awareness and tolerance of the space or gap, he further suggested that 'in distance and time between the going and coming of the primary object, constitutes the "baptism" of space. If the infant can "contain" this space in the absence of his object, he is able to initiate and expand his sense of space and is able therefore to be separate' (ibid., p. 56). Grotstein's (1978) discussion on inner space is primarily the skin, and secondly the ability to separate that is similar to Milner's (1969) discussion referring to strength.

Looking at the components in the development of the capacity to experience inner space, it is vital to look at what in my view is not described in psychoanalytic literature on resilience as inner space or lack of it that is the emptiness and vulnerability. I think the experience of empty space may be there from the start and this experience of the patient in transference may reach the analyst's experience in countertransference. This corresponds with Kernberg's (1975) account of extreme schizoid emptiness, in which patients sooner or later culminate in the psychotic loss of the experience of inner emptiness. This is particularly the case when the patient has lost the experience of having a body, hence inner and outer emptiness fuse to become a void and in transference the patient no longer able to experience the self and the analyst as two individuals together. It is possible for patients to experience no one else existed in the group and have concrete phantasies of all sorts in a void in the space. This psychic space or lack of it is linked with dissociation.

Free association

Free association the process of free association is one of the primary methods of working psychoanalytically. It helps the patient to recognise and overcome possible innate resistance which may be exhibited as hostility towards the analyst. The rationale is to defuse the superego and moderate its efficiency as a screening mechanism, so material which would otherwise be repressed is allowed to filter through to the patient consciousness. This will provide space to work through strengthening the ego. Freud (1912b) evolved the technique of free association as an alternative to hypnosis in view of its perceived fallibility. He found with free associations patients could make progress and come to terms with important memories while conscious. He remarked that despite patients' effort to remember, certain defences and resistance can prevent free association to the painful memories, as certain painful and traumatic memories are totally repressed, and prohibited in the conscious sphere of the mind.

Dreams

Dreams and the association by the mean of interpretations is an additional main technique in the practice of psychoanalysis. The rationale for dream analysis is similar to that of free association. Working with dreams, linking its associations to the past and present in transference helps the patient to gain insight and enhanced ego function. In some cases when the patient have and can clearly recall the dream of nightmare help us as the analyst to work with material that previously was denied. Dream interpretations as a method of intervention can successfully enhance a better self-knowledge for the patient presenting the dream in the group as well as augmenting recovery for the group as whole and creating better connectedness.

It is important to mention here that for refugee patients specifically those involved with politics, dreams and free association are of particular importance as these patients are usually motivated by a strong super-ego which of course functions less effectively in sleep, as well as in free association. It is also important to note that there is a distinction between the manifest content of a dream, what the dream appeared to be about, and its latent content, the unconscious, repressed needs or desires.

The interpretation of dreams, slips of tongue and free-associations will leads to the participants unconscious repressions engendering undesirable neurotic symptoms. With analyst who is facilitating possibility for impression and feeling freely patients can become conscious of unresolved conflicts buried in the deep unconscious mind. When successful, this process leads to sublimation as patients discovering the function is on superego and the social constraints. Such a discovery helps patients to decide to satisfy own instinctual drives. In all of these the group is moving by a kind of catharsis, the process of conveying to the repressed emotions, complexes, and feelings, in an effort to identify and release them.

Mourning

Referring to *Mourning and Melancholia*, Laplanche and Pontalis (1973) described mourning as follows:

> Intrapsychic process, occurring after the loss of a loved object, whereby the subject gradually manages to detach himself from this object … a psychical phenomenon treated traditionally as a gradual and apparently automatic attenuation of the suffering caused by the death of a loved one.
>
> (Laplanche & Pontalis, 1973, p. 485)

Freud (1917) initially indicated that mourning comes to an important and 'spontaneous end', when the survivor has detached emotional ties to the lost object and reattached the free libido to a new object – thus forbearing comfort in the form of a substitute for what has been lost. This assumes a view of subjectivity and object-love, and optimism for post-war recovery that Freud articulated in *On Narcissism* (Freud, 1914a). In this work, Freud defended against the cultural repression of loss by defining mourning as an essential process, theorising the psyche as an internal space for grief work, and bringing a discussion of bereavement into the public domain. He later (Freud, 1923) redefined the identification process previously associated with melancholia as an integral component of mourning. By viewing the character of the ego as a melancholic formation, he identified similarities between the two responses to loss, suggesting that mourning and melancholia necessitate similar symptoms. Freud indicated that 'profoundly painful dejection, cessation of interest in the outside world, loss of the capacity to love, inhibition of all activity' (Freud, 1923, p. 244) and 'reaction to the loss of a loved person, or to the loss of some abstraction which has taken the place of one, such as one's country, liberty, and ideal, and so on' (ibid., p. 243) can lead to melancholia. In contrast to the predominant feelings of love that made the completion of mourning possible, melancholic grief has ambivalent feelings of love and hate for the other. This ambivalence stems from 'a real slight or disappointment coming from this loved person' (Freud, 1917a, p. 249). Also 'each single one of the memories and expectations in which the libido is bound to the object is brought up and hyper-cathected, and the detachment of the libido is accomplished in respect of it ... when the work of mourning is completed, the ego becomes free and uninhibited again' (ibid., p. 245). Freud's description of primary narcissism, like his theory of object love, implies that we love others less for their uniqueness and separateness, and more for their ability to contract our own profusion that is to represent and reflect on the part of our self we have invested in them. This means people we love are replaceable and it is not possible to differentiate exactly how other they are. It is this model of the narcissistic subject that informs Freud's early morning theory, where the loss of a love objects is recognised as a transitory disruption of one's self as the mourner. This prompts us to give up the lost object by imagining that love for the other fundamentally derives from self-love, involving less grief for the leaving or death of an exceptional other, and more a process toward restoring a reliable economy of our self. By doing that we are retrieving a part of our self that has been projected to other for construction of our self image as a complete and autonomous being. Losing a loved one therefore threatens to break our imaginary psychic integrity. This explains why people cling to the lost object, given that acknowledging the loss would force us in our grief to recognise the full extent of what has been lost, that is to say an irrecoverable characteristic assign to the self, needed to our sense of coherent identity.

In response to the First World War, Freud returned to the subject of mourning in *Thoughts for the Times on War and Death* (Freud, 1915b) and *On Transience* (Freud, 1916b), in which he emphasised cultural ideals lost as a result of the war. He addressed the loss of 'so much that is precious in the common possessions of humanity' (ibid., p. 275), in seeking to dissolve the, 'mortification' and 'painful disillusionment' (ibid., p. 285), with which wartime violence and brutality is regarded. Further in *The Ego and the Id* Freud

(1923b), renounces the lost other, and incorporates the loss through a consoling substitute. The self is restored and the work of mourning brought to a decisive close, when the free libido has been reinvested in a new object. He formulated a perplexing dilemma in the human psyche; the eternal conflict between the dual instincts of Eros as the life instinct, and Thanatos as the death instinct. He referred to some aspects of the death instinct with superego aggression, implying that the superego was the agent of the death instinct in its aggressive need for punishment and its operative feeling is a punitive hatred, while other aspects of the superego were protective. This is helpful to understand in war, persecutions, political conflict and other forms of basic human right violations an individual may function on State superego and idealised as own ego and superego. This explains how during such conflicts the social superego is placed in the individual and how in turn the individual is positioned and acts in the social circumstances.

In line with Freud theory Melanie Klein (1946) termed projective identification, distinguishing between what is internal and what is external. She stressed that when diffusion or separation of the dual instincts occurred, aspects of aggression often become dominate, and that is the purpose of the ego to find objects for Eros or aggression either in phantasy or reality. This developed and was called projective identification by Klein (1946). Greenberg and Mitchell's description of Klein's theory is that

> projective identification was developed to describe extensions of splitting in which parts of the ego are separated from the rest of the self and projected into objects. ... Consequently, projective identification is a more interactional concept than the Freudian concepts of both projection and identification.
>
> (Greenberg & Mitchell, 1983, p. 128)

They further pointed out that

> for drive model theorists the repetition of painful experiences is more meaningfully understood in terms of instinctual conflict and subsequent anxiety and guilt ... The fact that retaliation is feared, even by the child who grew up in an objectively benign atmosphere, suggests that such fears are based on projected aggression.
>
> (Greenberg & Mitchell, 1983, p. 406)

Delusional projections

There are structural sets of internal needs which lead to projecting onto others the characters the person wants to see to will fulfil own needs. The reason this is important in working with people endured trauma and in particular refugees due to external atrocities. In delusional projections, the other is always seen through the distortion of emotionally overburdened internal relationships. At that juncture, it is possible 1. there will be no realistic perception of self as object to other. 2. The other cannot be perceived without adulteration by the self-internalised other that take account of the relationship with the other, which can be received in distorted form. 3. the more psychopathology, the less the person will be able to recognise others as they are. subsequently instead of the two individual units or people linked as a pair existing as a dialogue, it endures as projections.

Understanding these concepts is helpful and relevant in group work with traumatised refugees, given that becoming a refugee can involve losses of social world, as well as a total loss of the self or part of the self. Many refugees go through a consolatory or disturbing and model of mourning, with some force, as they have to acknowledge the socio-political morals and principles that are enmeshed with losses. Many who have lost their loved ones may also not go through consolatory mourning and not grieve and therefore exaggerate the pathology of melancholia that is a less loving, ambivalent, distractive, and violent grief. In a society with a cruel and repressive system many refugees come from, aggression can functions as mourning. Freud's mourning theory and further development are helpful to understand the private and public pain that some refugees may have been through. the issue of consolation, and apprehension of the problem of bereaved aggression, are integral psychoanalytic concepts needed in working with refugees.

However, it is important to note that Freud's changing ideas about mourning in the context of the Great War stand in contrast to wartime mourning practices in which groups of people from refugee communities represented their shared grief and found collective consolation through remembering undertakings conversant by classical religious and romantic traditions. In a sense Freud was writing about his own experience of trauma during WW1 and mourning was for him about loss of object. Freud (1914a) describes mourning as a mode of personal and social recovery and the process of reality testing with acknowledging that lost objects no longer exist. For a refugee this is applicable but might also be something much more. It is possible to be a total disruption, therefore the total loss of the self. Freud's (1914) early mourning theory indicates that when we reject the belief that everything has been lost, we are inspired by ourselves and as the result in our libido become free. We are then able to replace the lost objects with new ones that are as loving as the old ones, or even more precious. He later redefined the process of identification associated with melancholia as a fundamental part of both subject formation and mourning an object which was lost and has been set up again inside the ego that is an 'object-cathexis' that has been replaced by an identification. Freud (1917) recognised that he did not earlier appreciate the full significance of this process and did not identify how common it was. He suggested that the identification process he had previously linked to a pathological failure to mourn in fact makes available the only stipulation whereby the id leaves or give up its objects. Later, Freud (1926) in relation to his daughter's death nine years earlier came to think that even though the intensity of mourning does eventually fade, substituting the loss is impossible. So, even people are able to find a substitute for the gaping wound, it will differ from the person we have lost and mourning for. Freud (1917) discounts his theory and describes the enduring bonds of love that remain long after the other has departed, elaborating the identification process as a positive incorporation of the lost other. Laplanche (1999) critique of Freud's mourning theory addresses this affirmation of otherness in the self, of an enduring 'voice' belonging to the other, understood as 'related to the superego, but which is not entirely merged with it' (p. 254).

Object relations theory

The object relations theory is primarily concerned with love, especially the need for parental love, which is a development from drive theory and removed from the discharge mechanics of the libido. The term 'object-relations' refers to the self-structure we internalise in early childhood, which functions as a foundation for establishing and maintaining prospective relationships. Psychopathology is an expression of traumatic self-object internalisations from childhood acted out in our present relationships.

The works of Melanie Klein (1882–1960) elaborate on and extend Freud's original theory through interpretive perspectives, observations and clinical work with children which have a profound impact on object relations theory. Klein (1932) saw connections between young children's coping strategies in play, and psychotic symptoms. She observed processes in pre-oedipal children that were very similar to oedipal conflicts, and applied her practice and theory of working with children in her work with psychotic adult. Klein (1940) emphasised that all adults at some level hold on to such psychotic processes, and are involved in an endless struggle to cope with paranoid anxiety and depressive anxiety. Her method of practice involved of using deep interpretations which she felt communicated directly with the unconscious, thus bypassing the ego defences. Her view on love and hate indicating that the other we hated is also the other that we love and the line of reasoning that the depressive position occurs when we can take in the other as a whole object. This can lead us to feel the need to attack, can also lead to taking in and tolerating more pain, which is linked to ambivalence that we can love and hate a person and still have a relationship. In this context the depressive position is reached when we realise that our love and hate are directed to the same object when the unconscious impulses to repair objects felt to have been damaged by destructive attacks of hate that is inherent in depressive feeling. Klein assumed that anxiety originated in aggression fundamentally innate and grounded in the projection of the death instinct outwards from the self. This stress on anxiety, internal danger threats and the workings of the death instinct were to have important consequences for her formulation of the concept of phantasy and the nature of creativity. Klein (1946) was interested in schizoid phenomena and developed ideas of the 'paranoid-schizoid position'. Paranoid schizoid and depressive positions concepts provide basic landscapes of our everyday thinking, depending on a model of the mind where our rational and irrational superego and id are functioned by our ego to sustain peace, a notion that we are in our inner world playing between splitting, projective identification and persecution on the one hand, and integration, depressive anxiety and reparation on the other. In Freud's model, the irrational goes on one side of the line, and the rational on the other, while Kleinian prototype they are muddled, therefore we constantly between these two basic positions managing our paired emotions of love and hate, envy and gratitude.

With regard to mourning, Klein (1952a) indicated that mourning involves repetition of the emotion experienced during the depressive position. Under the stress of fear of loss of the loved m/other, the infant struggles with the task of integrating the inner-world of building up secure good objects within the self. Klein (1946) thought that the ego is unable of splitting the object internally and externally, without a parallel splitting taking place within the ego. So the main processes which come into play in idealisation are operative in hallucinatory gratification and splitting of the object and denial of both frustration and of persecution. The frustrating and persecuting object is held apart from the idealised object. The bad object is denied, as is the whole situation of frustration and the psychic pain to which frustration gives rise, which is bound up with denial of psychic reality. The denial of psychic reality becomes possible through strong feelings of omnipotence, an essential characteristic of the early psyche. Omnipotent denial of the existence of the bad object and of the painful situation is in the unconscious to annihilation by the destructive impulse. It is not an object that is denied and annihilated, but also the object relation, a part of the ego, from which the feelings towards the object not originated, but are also denied and annihilated. This is important in working with refugees who have various ways of splitting the ego and internal objects, which results in the feeling that the ego is in pieces, leading to a state of disintegration and total disturbance, often called dissociative disorder and also depersonalisation. This I also find helping to recognise the mechanism of survivor guilt that many clinicions considered as common presentation in refugees narratives

As I discussed in details in the group chapter, I think it is important to note the work of Bion (1897–1979), which significantly advanced and re-conceptualised Klein's thinking. Bion (1957) indicated that envy involves 'attacks on linking,' projected to cut off problematic object relationships, but which, in the end, lead to a destruction of one's good objects. He introduced the very useful concept of 'containing' anxiety in the mother and infant, or patient and analyst, relationship. Drawing on this fundamental insight, Bion (1957) believed that one of the central tasks of the psychoanalyst is to contain the anxiety of the patient through the use of projective identification, in which the patient projects intolerable anxious feelings onto the analyst who in turn contains and interprets back to the patient the experience in a cohesive and manageable form. This I find to be relevant to many patients who have a high level of anxiety and are in constant need of a containing environment and contained relationship.

In summary, in my view after Freud Klein (1946) transformed the oedipal drama by identifying the m/other as central and thus playing a vital role in object relations theory. Her theory of splitting and projective identification concepts of difference and otherness as enemy is relevant psychopathology. Bion's (1957) development of Klein's theory into what he called the 'container' and the 'contained' offers some way out of the psychic dangers of projective identification by suggesting that we may be able to access our internal psychic world as a transformative power to combat violence both internally and externally. Object relations as the relational model, which accounts for the distortion of objects by pointing to the inherent difficulty of the search for relatedness, is the most useful theory in working with refugees. While object relations theory is a particularly effective approach when working with refugees, it is important to note that by limiting the family structure to nuclear family members does not take into consideration the fundamental roles played by extended family members in some refugee cultures, where individualist tendencies are almost not exist. The object relations view developed within the context of the western family structure, in which by in large the mother and father set up their family unit in a new location. To the author's knowledge, there is no psychoanalytical study of extended family systems in which there are multiple carers or mothering and fathering figures relating to the child's early life, and how the developmental process may differ in such instances. In some cultures and family systems women have a rota for breast feeding each other's children.

Chapter 7

Intercultural approaches for groups

Resilience and vulnerability are important factors in every person's mental health, and especially for refugees and asylum seekers. Resilience quality or lack of it in individual patients is a sign of trauma and adversity. Mental health or ill is the key element to understanding the impact of inequalities on health and other area of the refugee and asylum seekers life. It is abundantly clear that the chronic stress of struggling with material disadvantage is intensified to a very considerable degree where people live with inequality and are marginalised with the societies they are living. The relationship between inequality and poor health is of course not just issues for refugee and asylum seekers and interrelated within the social hierarchy and is global, even developed nations. The emotional and cognitive effects of high levels of differentiation in people social status are profound and far reaching. The distributions of economic and social wealth and resources as well as freedom are foundation of ill or health for general populations. The importance of the social and psychological dimensions of material deprivation and poverty are important factors for the practice of intercultural psychoanalysis as it informs past and current indicators of the patient as well as capturing missing dimensions.

For these reasons, levels of mental distress among refugee and asylum seekers, indeed other marginalised communities need to be understood less in terms of individual pathology and more as a response to relative deprivation and social injustice, which erode the emotional, spiritual and intellectual resources essential to psychological wellbeing. While psycho-social stress is not the only route through which disadvantage affects outcomes, it does appear to be one of the central one. The health-damaging behaviours and violence can lead to strategies of vulnerable and hopeless individual to outburst of anger and despair related to in the face of multiple problems such as occupational insecurity, poverty, debt, poor housing, exclusion and other indicators. These problems impact on intimate relationships, the care of children and care of the self, including the general population with the highest prevalence of anxiety and depression and post trauma symptoms.

Looking back, I realise that it is now over two decades since I established the first group at the Refugee Therapy Centre as intercultural psychoanalytic

DOI: 10.4324/9781003401322-8

groups. I feel both joy and sadness when I contemplate the progress, the changes the many has been positive with some negative.

In my view the intercultural therapeutic intervention not just for trauma, but in general need to be developing in the changing world and relentlessly changing environment in terms of physical, technological, power and human dimensions. One of the major reasons for the velocity in the changing world is increased of people stress due to the social inequality and the ongoing reduction of resources in financing health and social care. Search for funding and the search for implications of intercultural approach in my view need to become one of the priorities for restorative justice in society, including health and social care in general and mental health specifically, to keep the limited resources to be used best. As a clinician working with the most traumatised people due to war, social oppressions, persecutions, imprisonments, torture and other human right violations, it is vital to think and reflect how can we work effectively within such conditions we are exposed to in the new world. How can we challenge what we take to be the standards and medians for a health and wellbeing? How can we find time and space to think objectively while under pressure, and discover the potential for creative engagement with others in our separate and joint tasks, recognising and valuing our differences and commonalities? If we can bring ourselves to think and reflect on our own life and our differences and accept them as reality, with that knowledge we could have intercultural relations with our patient.

Much of intercultural psychoanalytic therapeutic approach in general and specifically in the group and its progress will result in understanding the triggers for the multiplicity of recurrently changing emotional state of mind and viewpoints that are stimulated in relationship with each other in the group, indeed with the analyst. It is of paramount importance for patient progress to understand and learn to recognise feelings toward the analyst stems from unconscious. Some of these feelings may be embarrassing, irrational or hostile, but is important to verbalise them. On the surface patient inner mechanisms work may be on defence against progress as a way of protections from painful areas without conscious knowledge. Such reluctance and disinclination to explore deeper takes the manifest form of negative feelings against the analyst, to other group members, or both. These feelings by and large based on the person earlier experiences, thoughts and feelings toward parents or primary carer. In such instances patients' reactions may be strong and it is our responsibility as the analyst to facilitate an environment for patient to gain insight and work through. Sometimes, there may be need for reminding the group boundaries and participants about the importance of self-discipline, especially when hostile feeling is expressed in the group to each other, not to give in to such feelings. In these types of situations doubts may come for particular patient. He/she may feel not benefiting being in the group and thinking there is no progress in the group. The periods of standstill or setbacks are inherent occurrences in psychoanalysis and in some ways in other type of therapeutic approach. Most often these periods are part of therapeutic process and progress and will be for limited duration. Old patterns of feeling of obstinate and persistent will without doubt influence progress and can temporarily create many ups and downs in the patients. Often an old pattern will recur when a hidden wound within patient unconscious is touched upon in the process of therapeutic encounter or specific interpretations, or when the next step forward seems too frightening to the person. Nonetheless, these processes are important and provide valuable insights and further progress. Dissociations and resistance will be part of patient defences in analysis, including group psychoanalysis that I discussed in more details in another chapter.

As analyst it is important for us to ensure that patient is aware of the process and encouraged to express feelings toward analysts or fellow group members without fears. Learn to observe others emotional reactions. The significance of these reactions may appear in what is said, but more importantly how it is said. The analyst may notice when a patient is acting out an emotion, that is, when the emotion can only be finds expression in action rather and not in verbalisation in that particular instance. This might be, for illustration, be turning back on and ignoring the analyst or group members, or constantly interrupting others, or knowingly make false and malicious statements about another group member or the analyst with intentions to hurt them, or falsely claim affection for analyst or another group member to gain attentions and creating grouping within the group. Understanding the feelings underlying such actions, that are often unconscious, will facilitate greater insights into one's feelings and behaviours participating in the group and this is best done by interpretations. We know that people emotional structure and behaviours patterns have been shaped and ingrained in early developments from early childhood, thus, the timely and continued interpretations over an extended period usually will result in lasting changes. An important part of the psychoanalyst's job is upon finding the relevant unconscious conflicts and motivations that may present in transference to us as the analyst as well as other group members. By providing appropriate interpretations, patients can gain insights related to the past and its meaning in present life, by gaining new insight each person can apply them constructively in the day-by-day potential struggle and encounter against the old patterns, feeling content with a better intellectual understanding of any conflict, and try to make a conscious effort to remember any insights gained.

During the process of therapeutic interactions in the group, I over and over observed while patient feel and accept the positive changes and better insight and self-awareness, also, may feel lose. Most of the time in the beginning people present what we understand as psychosomatic pains, symptoms usually shown in the body, mainly back, knee and head, especially people who have endured torture and other forms of human rights violations. As therapy progresses and person can feel psychologically better, the bodily pains will subside. We need to give attention, in response to this change, even we see it as positive some patients may consider ending therapy and leaving the group. It is vitally important while considering leaving which is their right, we propose a period of ending, so, patient can listen to the analyst and other participants view to understand whether the uncomfortable or unfamiliar feelings of changes is temporary or can be more permanent, or actually the deep structural changes have been achieved which is positive and worth continue making more changes. In some circumstances resistive forces can be the underlying cause for the feeling psychologically well and strong and, more often than not, unconscious resistance to predicted projected anxiety and not necessary the improvement to the level to make decision to leave. The analysis remain unfinished if a participant contemplates the possibility of leaving that can be unconsciously relating in avoiding deeper painful feelings not yet emergent and that are now ready to surface. It is important to explore in the group before a patient decide to leave to ensure time is right of the patient.

In groups I developed at the Refugee Therapy Centre, I introduced a system that in practice I find the outcome to be positive. From the beginning I set three particular times for people who decide to leave, April, before spring break, July before summer break and December before winter break. I proposed to group from the beginning that we all know separations might be difficult, so, if you decide to leave for any reason you have, it is good to give some notice and leave just before any of three breaks during the year. For members who have no intention to leave, automatically commit to remain participant until the next break. This was helpful and we have good results. Almost 100% it worked for individual and all group to determine whether this wish or thought of leaving the group is a result of resistance to further change or a justified decision based on the solid ground of mental health achievement. Most of the time it was the latter. Member wants to study, or find a job and wanted to be positive contributor to society. One of the reason, I initially thought about potential uprooted leaving was based on the fact that many individuals in thus groups I have worked with and presenting in this book forced to leave their home and familiar environment without prepare plane, just to survive atrocities and to rescue their life and did not have opportunity to say goodbye to their loved one, and in many instances the leaving could not be shared with closest to protect them and to keep themselves safe until they reached a safe place.

It is particularly important for refugees or others whose forced to leave their country to explore ending therapy within the group and discuss it in a few sessions. This is of great consequence for the person leaving, indeed other participants to have opportunity to end and say goodbye. This process was not easy for the group, but it would provide opportunity for group members to have choice and to grieve and to celebrate different chapter in a member life. On many occasions it was challenging to deal with the grief in the group.

Some members more resistance to be vulnerable were making all sort of proposals such as inviting the leaving person to come to the group once a month or every three months. We know dealing with the trauma and atrocity is not without psychological hazard. As the analyst, I with gentle interpretations involve a deliberate use of myself as an instrument helping patients to grieve and to let go. My countertransference as a living response to the patient's emotional state at any given moment, played an empathic attunement to the patient's experience of trauma and not having a choice was central to my interpretations and having choices. I then present my gratification and contentment as the analyst to the leaving member who provides us all in the group a process of discussions before leaving for a good fairwell.

Recognising, reflecting to understand and monitor my countertransference in working in the group with people endured trauma was an intrinsic interactive perspective providing analytical tool and working model in terms of manifestation, source, function, impact and use. Having highlights the importance of the countertransference, my closure also was an important matter and I needed to be careful to make appropriate decision for disclosure of my countertransference consideration and its suitability in order to prevent any destruction to the group encounter and relationship. I recognise that I need to be patient to learn and able to differentiate countertransference for potential vicarious traumatisation or what is termed as secondary traumatic stress, burnout and compassion fatigue that will be hazarders in the group. I learned some characteristic differences between trauma groups and other psychoanalytic groups and the analyst countertransference. Trauma as content is major in such group, the anger, defence, dissociations and resistance as protection can limit the analyst response, in order not to cause further stresses for patients. The assessment and monitoring of our countertransference is significantly important, so does the risk of vicarious or secondary traumatisation and compassion fatigue. Understanding trauma is important for the group analyst leading a trauma group. Theory and what we have learn in our training can help us as a means to normalise and contain anxiety about what is observed and what can be expected of patients in any given moments in the group on the road to recovery.

One of the important matters I discussed in the chapter on trauma is the need to bear in mind the diagnostic criteria of the post-traumatic stress in the *ICD-10* as well as *DSM-5* (American Psychiatric Association, 2013). I will here, only focus on the latter on the diagnosis of Posttraumatic Stress Disorder (309.81) (ibid., pp. 467–468). Patients who may experience at least one of the following intrusive symptoms associated with the traumatic event can be diagnosed as suffering from PTSD. These usually are unexpected or expected reoccurring, involuntary, intrusive and upsetting memories of the traumatic event, the repeated disturbing dreams or nightmares where the content of the dreams is related to the traumatic event. In *DSM-V*, the American Psychiatric Association revised the PTSD diagnostic criteria.

PTSD is included in a new category, 'Trauma- and Stressor-Related Disorders'. PTSD symptoms are generally grouped into four types: intrusive memories, avoidance, negative changes in thinking and mood, and changes in physical and emotional reactions. Symptoms can vary over time or vary from person to person. DSM-5 also include the addition of two subtypes of PTSD in children younger than 6 years and PTSD with prominent dissociative symptoms (either experiences of feeling detached from one's own mind or body, or experiences in which the world seems unreal, dreamlike or distorted). The stages of PTSD are considered to be:

- *Impact* or *emergency* stage. This phase occurs immediately after the traumatic event.
- *Denial* stage. Not everybody experiences denial when dealing with PTSD recovery.
- *Short-term recovery* stage. During this phase, immediate solutions to problems are addressed.
- *Long-term recovery* stage.

Common symptoms of PTSD are the following:

- vivid flashbacks (feeling like the trauma is happening right now);
- intrusive thoughts or images;
- nightmares;
- intense distress at real or symbolic reminders of the trauma; and
- physical sensations such as pain, sweating, nausea or trembling.

NICE guidelines planning treatment and supporting engagements when discussing treatment options with people with PTSD and their family members or carers are to give them information about any proposed interventions, including:

- their aim, content, duration and mode of delivery;
- the likelihood of improvement and recovery;
- what to expect during the intervention, including that symptoms can seem to get worse temporarily; and
- that recovery is more likely if they stay engaged with treatment.

The guidelines also advise the following:

- Take into account the person's preferences, any previous treatment, associated functional impairment and coexisting conditions.
- Take into account any social or personal factors that may have a role in the development or maintenance of the disorder, such as childhood maltreatment and multiple traumatic experiences.

- Be aware that people with PTSD may be apprehensive, anxious, or ashamed. They may avoid treatment, believe that PTSD is untreatable, or have difficulty developing trust. Engagement strategies could include following up when people miss appointments and allowing flexibility in service attendance policies.
- For people with PTSD whose assessment identifies a significant risk of harm to themselves or others, establish a risk management and safety plan (involving family members and carers if appropriate) as part of initial treatment planning.

(NICE, 2018)

The essential feature of posttraumatic stress is the development of characteristic symptoms following exposure to an extreme traumatic stressor involving direct personal experiences of an event that involves actual or threat of death or serious injury, or other threat to one's physical integrity; or witnessing an event that involves death, injury or a threat to the physical integrity of another person; or learning about unexpected or violent death, serious harm, or threat of death or injury experienced by a family member or other close associate. The person's response to the event must involve intense fear, helplessness, or horror (or in children, the response must involve disorganised or agitated behaviour). The characteristic symptoms resulting from the exposure to the extreme trauma surely will include persistent experiencing of the traumatic event as well as avoidance of stimuli associated with the trauma and numbing response or reaction or in contrast increased arousal. Traumatic experiences render people helpless, overwhelming sense of losing control, connection, and meaning. When the overwhelming force is that of other human beings such as torture or other forms of human right violations like child abuse or war the trauma is specifically damaging as compared with when the force is found in nature. The Three Symptom Clusters that Judith Herman (1992), in her seminal work on *Trauma and Recovery*, considers that a person's response to trauma is usually manifested in three symptom clusters. These symptoms reflect the fact that each component of the ordinary response to danger, having lost its utility, persists in an altered and exaggerated state long after the actual danger is over.

- Hyperarousal: 'The persistent expectation of danger.' There is an inability to sleep, relax, eat; emotional liability (the person is easily upset, frightened or angered); intolerance for the stimulation of people, crowds, television; panic and anxiety attacks, dissociative symptoms.
- Re-experiencing: 'The indelible imprint of the traumatic moment.' There are intrusive images, thoughts, memories, nightmares, and flashbacks.
- Constriction: 'The numbing response of surrender.' There is little or no affect, the person can't feel, can't cry, and can't remember. There is an avoidance of anything associated with the trauma or anything emotional

or upsetting; an avoidance of social connections, places and things of former interest; an overall disinterest in life's events or in the future.

And three-stage process of healing and recovery according to Herman (1992) as the core experiences of psychological trauma are disempowerment and disconnection from others. As such, recovery from trauma is based on empowerment and the creation of new connections with self, the other, one's belief system and the world. Herman offers a three-stage process of healing and recovery. Using this as a basis, a group analyst in trauma group would consider recovery in terms of the following:

1 *Establishing safety*: Restoration of physical safety by attention to physical healing, sleeping, eating and environmental needs. Normalising posttraumatic stress (PTS) symptoms, establishment of trusted places and people, management of exposure and distance from the trauma. (In group, safety is developed by the presence of analyst, empathic attunement, established frame, symptom management, pacing, and containment).
2 *Remembering and mourning*: Involves the retrieval, reconstruction and transformation of traumatic memories by sharing them in a protective relationship. All traumas involve loss. The unanticipated death of a loved one involves assault and then loss. Grieving is a unique process of slowly transforming loss by connection and permission to remembering.
3 *Reconnecting*: Involves the movement from isolation and helplessness to connection with life, self, and others by use of therapeutic relationships, support networks, coping skills, qualities of resilience such as creativity, intelligence, sense of humour, spirituality, new meanings in life- sometimes a survival mission.

There has been considerable recognition of the viability of group intervention for people who have same or similar traumatic experiences including those endured torture and other forms of human right violations. Similarity of other group shared type of trauma such as combat veterans, adult survivors of child abuse, domestic violence, refugees, asylum seekers, people experiences torture, parents of adolescence and many others. Group interventions are effective in addressing PTS syndromes of trauma because they share key features that build a safe and respectful therapeutic environment, but from psychoanalytic view, we surely as analysts need to visit and revisit countertransference.

Freud (1910b) originally considered countertransference to be the analyst's unconscious reaction to the patient's transference and was viewed as a hindrance, something to be analysed away. Evolved psychoanalytic understanding as a result of the contributions of analysts such as Heimann (1950), Racker (1968) and Kernberg (1965) reconsidered countertransference as a natural and normal development. In their totalistic view, countertransference includes all the analyst's responses (pathological or appropriate) as a source of significant understanding of the patient in the ongoing process. Racker's differentiation of countertransference into concordant (identification with the patient's ego) and complementary (identification with some split off part of the patient) furthered the analyst's understanding and use of counter-transference. It was Racker (1968) who recommended that the analyst first develop an understanding of the patient's internal process in the here and now and then use the countertransference in formulating appropriate reactions.

The countertransference always includes conscious and important elements of unconscious response and feelings, as well as the verbal and non-verbal reaction to and interactions with the patient based on our theoretical perspective, training, experience, our age, gender, marital status, and race or ethnicity, our characteristic personality, history, current life events, and our psychological and physical needs. The interactive characteristic of transfer-ence-countertransference enhance and increase to the intersubjective context will generate constructs by the interaction of the analyst's total counter-transference and that of the total patient transference as parallel dynamics, indeed similarly parallel with other participants in the groups

There is always possible for us as analyst to have recurring, repetitive or cyclical countertransference unwittingly enacting on our own unresolved life issues, not necessarily relevant to the patients presenting issues. Reparative countertransference in the group, where analyst experiences a replay of own past, and sometimes with interpretations unconsciously attempts to repair own wounds not relevant to the group member. There is also a situation where our countertransference corresponding with the same feelings as the group members. In such transference-countertransference we are mirroring the group. This is similar to what Racker (1968) refers to as 'concordant countertransference'. Sometimes complexity may be presented in counter-transference in groups where we may face multiple and complex transference projections from different members in the group in a session. Compare to working with individual these are more challenging to deal with easily. In such encounters we need to give attentions to individuals as well as the whole group while making sure we are thinking and monitoring own counter-transferences. The impact of theory and styles of the way we work in mon-itoring and reflecting on countertransference in groups is much depends on a function of our understanding of psychoanalytic theory and clinical impli-cation, technique and style of interpretations. Theoretical orientation affects the countertransference and shapes our perceive transferences both with individual and in group setting. As an analyst we adhere to a juncture theory of mourning, it is therefore possible to trespass verbal and or nonverbal probabilities, enthusiasm or apathy in the group or towards individual parti-cipants for not moving on or letting go as we anticipated. If, we as the analyst contented with the use of unconscious associated with quantifiable probable matter, it is likely that we can encourage patients to focus more on the use of dreams in order to analyse unconscious context of particular presentations within the group. A close and similar experience between groups' participants and the analysts is an important component that needs ongoing reflections and discussions. This is vitally important especially when there are two analysts jointly facilitating a group, as to some degree there are transference-countertransference will also be between analyst to analyst within the group. The dynamics may occur between analysts, if we are not attended to that can become hazardous countertransference response to the group as a whole. I will consider those moments as fail because there are no analysts in the group, and everyone is patient.

It is important to note that two analysts working in partnership can be helpful and constructive in working with people endured trauma in the group because it allows for shared containing environment to facilitate painful narratives from patients' presentations that can creates difficult feelings. Where analysts working in pair, they can keep attentions on each other and provide affirmation for each other in the sessions and discussions and feedback after each group sessions. Such a co-analysis is particularly important for trauma groups as in such a group we may not be able at early stage follow the schema of developmental stages that we have learned in our training and employed in other groups. We know as a role of tam countertransference is important in ongoing analysis both in individual and groups, but it can be more complex and painful in working with people endured trauma and more so in groups.

The precarious frightening, terrorising and complex landscape of groups for people who have endured trauma require an experience analyst to identify, be familiar with and be able to accomplish complex dynamics. The analyst must be able to reflect and monitor own countertransference response to the traumatic material and the responses of individual group members and group as a whole, indeed the dynamics with the co-analyst. The analyst's responses are windows of opportunity for insight and compassion into the self and others' positive or negative past and present realities. There are of course no implicit and explicit boundaries those continuations of group need as long as initial explicit roles are maintained by members. The general group disclosure and communications norms for all members to each other need to be carefully monitored and evaluated by the analyst as the person who knows everyone. This ongoing monitoring and evaluations will focus on dynamic in the group and recognises issues that need addressing and interpreting patterns that have impaired interpersonal functioning, ego mastery and intimacy, in order to restore a sense of stability, security, ego capacity, as well as connection or reconnection with others to move towards a better future.

In the aftermath of tragedy or catastrophic event, the analyst immediate goal of responding is to establish safety through the creation of a 'containing and holding environment' (Winnicott, 1965) in the group. This sometimes can be achieved with normalisation of symptoms, the containment of affect, attentiveness to evidence of physical or psychological decompensation, empathic attunement, active listening, visual monitoring of the verbal and non-verbal communications responses of each member to the analyst and members to each other, and balancing anger, grieve, irritations, frustrations, aggravations, stimulations and motivations to share as well as permission to just observe.

As the analyst I with an awareness of the devastating and incapacitating explanation of trauma and grief can assimilates a safekeeping and direction as I discussed and set up in initial meeting as the group role and boundaries of the group. By and large in psychoanalytic group silence plays a great part of the analysis but in group for people endured trauma long silence can create uncomfortable feelings as well and unstructured response, rigid or demanding response may not be helpful in facilitating a safe and containing group. While respecting the individual's timeline, as analyst we need to consider when to highlight and accentuate differentiation as well as historical perspective, self-introspection and regenerated mastery in a heterogeneous group. In some situation the group can be conceptualised as the substance of an internalised structure facilitating the first step in connecting again with the world that may have been lost as the result of trauma. I think, this approach I consider intercultural or relational in working in the trauma group will better create and support cohesion. So, for patients leaving the group will not be scary or complicated and once again the individual can build the strong bond inherent in a mutual experience prior to the effect of trauma.

Intercultural Psychoanalytic approach in my view and experiences continues to make important contributions to basic clinical understanding of adaptive and maladaptive psychological development. It is a useful method of clinical intervention to examine personality development and for understanding various forms of psychopathology as deriving from disruptions of normal developmental processes. Indeed, it is helpful for conducting epistemological research on the therapeutic process in both individual and group therapeutic interventions. Psychoanalytic thought, in some of its manifestations, holds a strong capacity to view the operation of both the internal and external, indeed emotional and social world of the person. In the life of traumatised refugees, emotions are at times overwhelming to the point of leading to precipitating self-destructive behaviour or enactments of violence. They seep through to the surface and influence social experience, in situations such as internal fear, intense ambivalence and collapse of external disintegration or a pervading sense of immobility in the face of palpable danger. Working with refugee patients, the focus will primarily be on developing awareness of vulnerability and identify resilience that may have been lost, both building on inner strength and a capacity for holding what is thought to be uncontainable. Within the context of therapeutic intervention, not to consider the innate and developing but often covert resilience of the person's internal world is like attending to the external presentation of a person without considering what the person feels inside. Both are necessary components of the therapeutic task that is the psychoanalytical practice.

In my view, what is required in group therapy with traumatised people is analytic thinking as dynamic and variable of each person within the group, with the aim to consider the internal and external world, the good and the bad, the strength and the weakness, the past and the future as well as the immediacy of the present that is evident in the real life of a refugee and in transference within therapeutic encounter. Therefore, the focus should be on three areas of object relation as well as reconstruction of history and the personality development of the patients. Freud (1905a, 1917b, 1937) pursued and searched for empirical and experimental confirmation of the validity of his discoveries. He emphasised the importance of establishing agreement between analytic reconstructions and the results of naturalistic child observation. The same objectives later led Stern (1985) to produce evaluations of infant research findings on analytic developmental propositions. The findings from the clinical work provide one kind of validation for psychoanalytic reconstructions, making it possible to provide a satisfactory level of inevitability in the attempt to integrate the patient's 'psychic truth' with 'actual' or historical truth (Freud, 1937a). The use of reconstruction is an important dimension of psychoanalytic technique that is regaining analytic attention to understand how an adult has remained a disturbed child with that particular psychopathology. The importance of reconstruction is imperative for restoring personality, continuity and cohesion and for explaining anxious and neurotic repetition compulsion as it has developed in past life and enacted in transference in the group.

This utilisation of reconstruction will be helpful to identify the linkage between historical events and the patient's intrapsychic structure, through the process of interpretation and response to the here and now, as well as the linkage between past and present, childhood and adult psychopathology. Reconstruction in the group may not always follow from the transference to the analyst but to other group participants; it is rather an inferential and integrative act from resistance and amnesia, which may also be the result of substance by chemical processes of memories and biological syntheses for missing memory and gaps in history as the result of trauma endured. However, the reconstructive integration identifies patterns and interrelationship aspects of patients' and the intrapsychic configurations consequences, rather than isolated conflicts and experiences. Therefore, developmental influences are more important than actual historical facts that contribute to the formation, testing, and validation of psychoanalysis.

I find Henry Ezriel (1956) writing in group helpful, though not always practical in my group works completely. He refers to his analytic group work as testing of psychoanalytic theory and practice. His work in the group set-ting, tended to be as if he was working with one patient, and to seek unifying themes, assumptions, and trends in the interaction of the members. He restricts his activity as analysts to two basic tenets: first, everything the patients say or do is related to the analyst; second, the only intervention of the analyst is to interpret, and with each interpretation to focus on and strengthen the view that all intrapsychic and interpersonal behaviour of all the patients is always analyst-oriented, always transferential. Ezriel (1956) later discussed that in his group work he 'refrained from making and refer-ence to the past and used solely here and now interpretations' (p. 48). He emphasised that a strict here and now approach will allow the experimental study of the behaviour of an individual in the psychoanalytic intervention. He concludes that 'a here and now approach without reference to the patient's past, overcomes objections which are commonly brought against the possibility of using the psycho-analytic session as an experimental situation in which hypotheses about human behaviour can be tested' (ibid., p. 48)

The therapeutic effectiveness of the interpretation and reconstruction of repressed past unconscious conflicts and trauma is important. Analytic lis-tening is an ongoing process, containing all the components of conflict and shaped in every moment by all patients and the analyst's conflicts as well as patients to each other in group interactions. The mutual responsiveness that develops in the group stems from complex conflictual object relationships that are no different from any other object relationship, in which transference and countertransference at all times simultaneously facilitates and interferes with the analytic work. Clinical process will show the usefulness to these and related phenomena, including the use of signal conflict, the benign vulner-abilities or at times negative transference and countertransference, the func-tion of countertransference structures, and the use of repetition compulsion, projections, introjections and projective identifications, shifting transferences and resistance, and the level of the object relationship continuously being created between analyst and participating patients.

I find Kohut's sense of self in *Restoration of the Self* (1977) also helpful in working with traumatised people in the group. It is helpful to think and identify which self or portion of the self my patient present in the group every given time. Kohut (1977) articulated that in all he had written on the psychology of the self, he had purposely not defined the self, knowing that some people would be critical of him about that omission. He described that it had become impossible to base his work on his predecessors because he would have been entangled in a 'thicket' of similar overlapping, or identical, terms and concepts which, did not carry the same meaning and were not employed as a part of the same conceptual context. He refers to a patient whose personality disturbance was marked by a vertical split in his person-ality. One fragment in his particular patient was characterised by a sense of superiority and messianic identification that result from a merger with his mother, who had idealised him and encouraged the grandiosity in him. Kohut (1977) also refers to cognitive impenetrability and says 'introspectively or empathically perceived psychological manifestations are open to us' (p. 311). For Kohut the self is 'the way a person experiences himself as himself' (ibid., p. xv), a permanent mental structure consisting of feeling, memories and behaviours that are subjectively experienced as being continuous in time and as being 'me'. The self is also a 'felt center of independent initiative', an 'independent recipient of impression', the center of the individual's psychological universe (ibid., p. xv), and not simply a representation. He says 'our transient individuality also possesses a significance that extends beyond the borders of our life' (ibid., p. 180) and describes 'cosmic narcissism' which transcends the boundaries of the individual.

Along this line, I find Steiner (1993) articulations also helpful. He discusses that neurotic, perverse, borderline and psychotic patients all have narcissistic structures in their personality. He termed this 'psychic retreat' that are found with stuck patients, using the retreat in a transient and discretionary way:

> psychic retreats present major problems of technique. The frustration of having a stuck patient, who is at the same time out of reach, challenges the analyst, who has to avoid being driven either to give up in despair or to over-react and try to overcome opposition and resistance in too forceful.
>
> (Steiner, 1993, p. 131)

He argues that relief granted by the retreat is accomplished at the cost of isolation, stagnation and retraction that some patients may find it distressing while others accept the situation and relief but with despair associated with the failure to make real contact with the analyst or others. Sometimes the retreat is felt to be subjected to a malicious area and tedious nature:

> of the situation is recognised by the patient, but more often the retreat is idealised and represented as a pleasant and even ideal haven. Whether idealised or persecutory, it is clung to as preferable to even worse states which the patient is convinced are the only alternatives.
>
> (Steiner, 1993, p. 2)

Steiner (1993) talked about technical problems relating to the nature of interpretations and how they are likely to be received by the intensely frightened and hostile patient, who fears the abrupt and permanent loss of the 'psychic retreat'. He offers some ideas to analysts in their attempts to stay with the patient, and to understand more clearly what is going on at critically problematic points in the work. Steiner (1993) discussion assists me in recognising and understanding what is going on, and be more open to those moments in which I sometimes can be drawn into supporting role, rather than analyst role in response to the patient pathological organisation. His discussion on how and when to interpret the transference relationship of patients and to recognise when patient is ready to receive interpretations can be achieved, by careful observation and judgements of the patient's presentations.

Another of my useful learning comes from Tuckett (1994), who argues that validation in the clinical process depends on being as clear and specific as possible about the hypotheses. He discuss that in sessions interpretation mainly based on intuitive and 'quite spontaneous links arising from background orientations'. He emphasised the importance of the patient's and analyst's external reality and indicated that

> outside the session, a wider and more developed set of grounded hypotheses can be developed, intended to illuminate what seem to be the core issues that arise over time and the core problems suffered by the patient. Often such hypotheses will only be in the form of working orientations.
>
> (Tuckett, 1994, p. 1159)

He argues if the hypothesis can be conceptualised correctly into precise suppositions and theories explaining sets of observed events and predicting consequences, they can be evaluated by the analyst working with individual or in group. In Tucker view the validation of clinical process much depends on being clear and specific about our hypotheses, implying that while we make interpretations on intuitive hypotheses stem from background history and collections of observed clinical facts in the sessions interaction, it is good to also to give attention to patient experience and narrative of their interactions outside the session. Tuckett says:

> I think they can be more precisely thought through and then validated – that is, partially or wholly refined so that they 'fit' better and/or are rejected as not fitting, whether by the analyst working alone or in group discussion through the achievement of genuine consensus.
>
> (Tuckett, 1994, p. 1174)

It is important to recognise that the task of constructing and reconstructing the sense of the self in intercultural psychoanalytic therapy with people endured sever trauma in general and with refugee, we may encounter the problem of memory and its plasticity. In such circumstances when patient memory distorted, and there is the difficulty of reaching to real memory, there will be no clear narratives of events. We face with infantile amnesia that may not be clear whether it is the function of brain or the repressing mind. This makes the task of constructing meaningful narrations of histories challenging but it is possible that patient improve and remember in the group, especially with here and now transference, that will provide possibilities of working through. Focus on the here and now, is helping patients to find new strategies and new ways of interacting with the important people in their lives. By doing this, the memory and associations will come to explore the enigmatic and mysterious otherness of oneself which can play a great way for the reconstruction.

Here, to support these theories and discussions, I bring a very brief vignette of a patient. This young man of 23 was referred by his probation officer. He had committed a series of petty crimes over four years and showed no remorse every time he was arrested. In begging for assessment in the first session, he was extremely angry and wanted to justify his actions as retaliations against corrupt system that is 'killing him', he said. I gently stopped him and said he can tell me all about it, but can we start please by you telling me a little about yourself, your past prior to become refugee in the UK. To my surprise, he calmed down immediately and started. He said that he was sends to the UK at very young age and has been in different faster family until the age of 18. After the process of assessments, and prior to introducing the idea of group, we have met twice a week for a while. He had issues of not trusting others. initially he hold strong believes that I was using him and forcing him into therapy to get information from him. When he would get to this stage of doubt, he would miss a session without calling to cancel. I raised his lack of attendance and commitments in the next session. I said, he is not expected to trust me, but if he wants therapy to feel better, he need to give his time and commitments, otherwise we might just stop. He said he have other appointments when he missed our sessions. I propose that he bring his diary and by end of each session we could arrange and agree on the next session. He agrees and we had fallen into a routine where we could agree on the next appointment at the end of each session. This was the first time in my career to propose such arrangement, but I thought this young man need to feel in control. However, he then purposefully would propose a time that was clashing with my time. I felt this was his way of ensuring that he is the one keeping control. Although, I was receiving irritating behaviour and I felt under his thumb, theoretically, I thought that if I pointed out how he delay leaving sessions and acknowledged his probable provocations and motivations, he may feel attacked, and become more defensive, strike back and get even more paranoid. Having said this, I was aware of the little scared and abused boy who is painfully aware of his fears and I should try to find a way to help him to feel safer and make better use of sessions than just acting out. I reserved interpretations in that session for the following sessions. I then proposed planning our next meeting at the beginning rather than the end of the session. Initially he said that was ok, but as we were setting the next session he suddenly became irritated. He said I was manipulating him and he feels trapped, and that have to stop. I just said OK. I then said I am wondering whether he is scared to be controlled. He shouted that he knows he is being controlled. I said, if you are so strongly thinking this way, we need to think what brings you here. He said you should by now know that I am fearful of any types of commitment. I said, you never told me this, how should I know. You are coming to see me, there must be some part of you that can have trust on me and this process, but another part of you regret trusting me. It is not good state of mind to be in – is it? He said he didn't like being let down. So, he needs to protect himself and be careful to avoid trusting people and be rejected or betrayed. He said it is much better to be alone with your own pain, than sharing it with a person who does not care. I responded briefly and just said: I wonder how being so lonely may be like? We continue discussing his loneliness and fear of trusting people which was helpful to discuss his exaggeratedly critical superego as the barrier for him. He related to this positively and said he did not think about it this way before, but he now can see how he always feel troubled and preoccupied by what we call superego that originate from his early life of being considered to be deficient in being able and strong and remain feeble and weak. In this encounter, through projective identification, he could discharge his punitive and disciplinary superego and discover part of his ego as objects for relief. He then starts getting angry with himself for attacking and controlling himself for such a long time. He looked at me with strong gaze for the first time and said: I am pathetic, aren't I? I said, no, you are not, but I am taking this statement as you wanted me to help you, and you can trust me as a person who can help you to express feelings without being judged to find a way out of debilitating anger, anxieties and confusions. I then welcomed his new more lenient calmer being that allow us to focus on his real feelings and thoughts. He was pleasantly surprised. He said, 'You are OK, I think.'

I have presented this particular vignette using some clinical material of individual sessions to examine the patient's relating and the use of projective identification from object relations perspectives from intercultural perspectives with a young refugee. I also address patient presentations effect on myself and the analytic dyad. At times I clearly struggled to comprehend or appreciate the patient's projections whereas I was feeling enticed and pressed to act out the patient's unconscious object. I was aware that patient projective identification and his mental mechanism creates anger and my counter-transference feelings was an urge to argue with him, but I managed to control my frustration with him and my urge to reject him as unsuitable patient. Instead, I act as a translator for his unwanted feelings, toxic and horror depilating memory of traumatic experiences and his unwanted, confusing, or threatened parts of him that his ego was unable to cope with. By doing so the patient and I managed to gain enough understanding of what was going on, consciously and subconsciously. Patient was acting out in transference and I was seduced to enactment with my countertransference in the process and appropriate compliance to his need to be in control but my later interpretation help the patient to move on. These, I consider inter-cultural psychoanalytical approach. I do not stick to textbook only and can bring some flexibility that may be criticised by many psychoanalysts but result proved to be positive. I decided that he will benefit to be in the young men group. I invited this patient to join the group and he accepts. The brief narrative of our encounter in the process of assessment of this patient is representative of many others that I worked with.

Chapter 8

What is the group?

Freud could not have stated the necessary harmony of his thought any more forcefully, in relations to what the social scientists call 'the autonomy of the social', that social produce and reason operating at a different level from the psychological and authentically of group forces, even though they are inter-cede act of a go-between through the individual psyche. There is no relative autonomy, so, for Freud the central dynamic was the conceding of authority and conscience to the group analyst and the Oedipal dynamic. Bion (1959) while accepts Freud's claim that the family group is the basis for all groups but challenged Freud view on the group and group dynamics, indicating that Freud's view of the dynamics of the group seems to require supplementing rather than correction. He says Freud's view is not enough as its central position on group dynamics is engaged by primitive mechanisms as peculiar to the paranoid-schizoid and depressive positions. In other words, he suggests that it is not simply a matter of the incompleteness of the illumination provided by Freud's discovery of the family group as the prototype of all groups (Bion, 1967). Bion (1962a) suggests the Tavistock approach that focuses on primitive oedipal conflicts, part-object relations and psychotic anxieties while challenging Freud's view on the id, ego and superego, detailed in *The Future of an Illusion* and *Civilization and Its Discontents*, indicating what is happening in groups, and demonstrating id, ego and superego and the oedipal triangle and that is all a psychoanalyst need to know to asses and treat the individual, in groups and in society.

Bion's basic assumption contains features that correspond closely with primitive part objects that sooner or later turned to psychotic anxiety asso-ciated with these primitive relationships. These anxieties, and the mechanisms peculiar to them, have been presented by Melanie Klein (1952b). Her descriptions correspond with emotional states of the basic assumption group which aims different from the explicit task of the group and fitting to Freud's view of the group that although speak to the angle of psychotic anxiety, associated with phantasies of primitive part object. In Bion's (1967) view, what matters in individual and group behaviour is more primitive than the Freudian level of account and rationalisation. If we consider the ultimate

DOI: 10.4324/9781003401322-9

sources of our distress are psychotic anxieties, and much of what happens in individuals and groups is a consequence of defences construct against psychotic anxieties, so that we do not have to endure them consciously. The basic assumption distinctiveness appear far more to have the characteristics of defensive reactions to psychotic anxiety, and are not so much at variance with Freud's views as supplementary to them. In my view, it is necessary to work through both the stresses that appertain to family patterns and primitive anxieties of part object relationships. I consider the latter to contain the ultimate sources of all group behaviour. In this regards Bion (1965) impression is that the group approximates too closely, in the minds of the individuals composing it, to very primitive phantasies about the contents of the mother's body. The attempt to make a rational investigation of the dynamics of the group is therefore disturbed by fears, and mechanisms for dealing with them, which are characteristic of the paranoid-schizoid position. The analysis therefore cannot be carried without the stimulation and activation of those elements of the emotional situation that are in a close relationship associated to phantasies of the earliest anxieties that an individual in the group is coerced and compelled to. As the result whenever the pressure of anxiety becomes too great, individual in the group may take defensive action.

This psychotic anxieties in question can ultimately necessitate splitting and projective identification, part-object relations and punitive guilt feelings which are basic characteristic of the paranoid-schizoid position. These may alternate with whole object relations, concern for the object, and constructive or reparative guilt that are characteristics of the depressive position. Apparent difference between group and individual psychology is an illusion which emerges as unknown and impracticable to the individual in the group.

Joan Riviere (1952) suggests that from the very beginning of life, on Freud's own hypothesis, the psyche responds to the reality of its experiences by interpreting them or misinterpreting them in a subjective manner that augments its desire and preserves it from pain. This act of subjective interpretation of experience, which it carries out by means of the processes of introjections and projection, is called by Freud hallucination. It forms the foundation of what we mean by phantasy life of the individual. It is thus the form in which the real internal and external feelings and perceptions are interpreted and represented in the individual mind under the influence of the pleasure-pain principle. It seems as if one has to consider for a moment to see that, in spite of all the advances one may have made in adaptation of a kind to external reality, this primitive and elementary function of the psyche to misinterpretation and perceptions for person own satisfaction that retains the dominance in the minds.

In claiming that experiences are characteristically misunderstand and misapprehend at source and that misrepresentation to the point of hallucination is at the very foundation of occurrence or encounter Riviere (1952) view is that there are no misunderstand and misapprehend experiences, and there is no unbiased observation in life. Based on this view, it is possible to assume we don't start with absolute sense of facts and figures to be subjectively distorted. The experience can be drawn attention to and brought to light by irrational presentations in the processes. Hence, if we progress towards group therapy from this point of view from the start, we are perpetually taken in the medical model of psychosis. I come back to Bion who makes distinction between work groups, and what he called above 'basic assumption' groups, groups in the grip of a primitive unconscious phantasy. The first basic assumption he says is dependency that the group is convened in order to be sustained by the analyst on whom it depends for nourishment and protection. The second basic assumption is of pairing that involves feeling of belonging to an inspirational leader, especially one claiming to be or regarded as a saviour or liberator hope that will save the group.

Bion (1959) indicates that these are not conscious reactions as the participation in basic assumption activity requires no training, experience or mental development. It is prompt, unavoidable and instinctive. The basic assumptions involve a group analyst that could be an idea or inanimate object. The person as the analyst is therefore can be as much the creature of the basic assumption as any other individual member of the group. The loss of individual distinctiveness relates to the analyst of the group as much as to any participants. This defensiveness within the group processes can lead participants to regress with primitiveness. In such occurrences demonstrating the basic assumptions instantly emerge as formations of secondary to an early primal scene worked out on a level of part objects, and associated with psychotic anxiety and mechanisms of splitting and projective identification that can be characteristic of the paranoid-schizoid and depressive positions.

One of the successful examples of empirical psychoanalytic research is conducted by Henry Ezriel (1950) who managed methodical testing of psychoanalytic theory and practice in his analytic group work by focusing on here and now interaction in the group. His group setting approach tended to be as if he was working with one patient, seeking unifying themes, assumptions, and trends in the interaction of the members. He restricts his activity as a therapist to two basic tenets: (1) everything the patients say or do is related to the therapist; and (2) the only intervention of the group leader is to interpret, and with each interpretation to focus on and reinforce the view that all intrapsychic and interpersonal behaviour of all the patients is always therapist-oriented, and the interactions is always transferential.

Ezriel (1956) later explained that in his group work he 'refrained from making a reference to the past and used solely here and now interpretations' (p. 48). He emphasised that a strict here and now approach will allow the experimental study of the behaviour of an individual in the psychoanalytic group intervention. He take to mean that 'a here and now approach without reference to the patient's past, overcomes objections which are commonly brought against the possibility of using the psycho-analytic session as an experimental situation in which hypotheses about human behaviour can be tested' (1956, p. 48).

Here, I should briefly address the introjection and projection of individual in the group process that is vitally important. If not giving attention to these functions as an analyst we can develop fear and confusion within group encounter. In order to keep awareness on this aspects of the work, especially when working with people who have endured trauma of war, oppressions and human rights violations we need to be aware of the individual societal functions or lack of it as well as the culture. This is important as the social phenomena demonstrate a signal correspondence with psychotic processes in individuals that establishments are used to reinforce individual to comply with their rules and requirements. As a result, we can identify mechanisms of defence against anxiety, and that the mechanisms of projective and intro-jected identification operate in linking the individual manners in public and within the group interactions as well as with transference reactions to both analysts and other group participants. The projection and introjection pro-cesses therefor are based on social interactive processes. For example the oppressors, the liberals, the conservative policy and practice may work for short period but will reach to reactionary response from individuals and creates grouping as consequences of individual thinking and psychotic anxi-eties of institutional defences against people. This is logical reactions of human disposition for social change and reason that social trouble, irritant and struggle are become determined and tenacious against oppressive pro-blematic system. Changes in group processes can help restructuring of indi-vidual relationships at the phantasy level, with a consequential stipulation to indicate that one event is followed by another that can help individuals to accept and endorse changes in their existing patterns of defences against psychotic anxiety created by the social circumstances. Effective change in social interactions of individual is therefore requiring noticing, analysing and accepting the societal common anxieties and unconscious collusions under-lying the social defences determining phantasy of different types of social functions and relationships between people and those in power to govern. It is troubling to witnessing indifference, apathy, lack of interest and apprehen-sion that is exactly opposite attitudes of care and the provision of compas-sion, kindliness and functioning with responsibility. Sadly, the world we are living in is full of coercion, oppression, persecutions, torture, terrorisation, threats and fear to life that surely can lead to the psychotic anxieties and provoke rebellious grouping against those in power in society, leading to the people thinking that situations that exist is not sustainable anymore and causing difficulties for individual and at the society as whole in the deepest levels. The intensity and complexity of such anxieties are to be attributed most of all to the atypical irregular dimensions and incompetence of the work of those in power in society and therefore compels the individuals in society to form group to stimulate anew aptitude and competence contrary to those situations and the accompanying damages dictates to society as a whole. The embedded aim of such ingrained plans in the mind without the opportunity to discuss and developments of clear strategy, which operate within socio-political situations of society structurally, culturally and appropriate managements, for the eradication of oppressions and change as a real and tangible object that decrease each person involved to part-objects, going along towards sustainable free society for everyone life. There is a whole system of overlapping ways of evading the full force of the anxieties associated with death, the ones which lie at the heart of underlying unconscious forces from psychoanalytic perspectives that are far from being disentangled, by the very people created with dishonesty for benefit of self and for people with and around them. With an understanding of psychoanalysis and stimulating ideas into the unconscious of group dynamics specifically helps reaching to a deeper level of societal function and dysfunctions.

In this book I have focused upon a group of traumatised patients who have endured external trauma in adult life as a result of socio-political environment as well as whose biological needs for nurture and comfort. The ideas of setting up group for severely traumatised people were arose in working with mothers who were referred mainly by social services, solicitors or by court order as the result of child protection matters. Over and over again when I had the opportunity to meet these mothers individually and after developing some rapport with them to see them with their child, I observed mothers could not relate to the child beyond simple caretaking. They never smile at the child and when they encouraged in the session to play, they showed no pleasure from playing with them or in the child's emerging sense of aliveness. Not easy to witness and at times I was lost of what else I can do? It appears that the mothers' attachments to the child were to use the child as transitional objects. Physically together, but not able to be the child 'listening other', thus preventing child's adequate development of 'psychic space' and 'sense of self. Instantaneously, it was clear to identify that such children's emotional development became fixated in the constant in-between transition space. This fixation understandably led to specific types of character structure and ego defects. There seem to be extensive gaps in layers of the psychic apparatus which manifested themselves as defective modulating elements. These type of patients by and large shows behaviour, marked polarities of sane, sensitive, physically caring and rational. But, exhibiting a peculiar kind of fragmentation or dissociating in which connecting emotional bridges between care giver and child that were missing. There are many such patients amongst those who seek treatment with initial presentations of adult external trauma.

Based on these types of assessments and some level of interventions that was mostly related to the child protections and the safety of the child led me to thinking about setting up psychoanalytic woman groups. Why psychoanalytically when most of the contemporary literatures suggest other approach, mainly cognitive behaviour. Psychoanalysis acknowledged the conjectures of disassociation along the unconscious, but relates them differently to each other and traces mental life back to interplay between forces that prefer or hold back from one another. For example:

1   If one group of ideas remains in the unconscious, but there are conscious connotations – psychoanalysis does not have conjecture that there is a constitutional incapacity for fusion which may lead to particular types of dissociation that I am discussing in this study.
2   Psychoanalysis also maintains that the isolation and state of unconsciousness have been caused by an active opposition on the part of other groups as repression, and as something alike. This is an unaccommodating judgement in working with the types of trauma and types of dissociations that may be employed by a traumatised patient.
3   Psychoanalysis uses concepts of repressions which play important part in mental life. But, repression as precondition of the formation of symptoms presented by patients is not enough as it can frequently fail in assessment and treatment of trauma patients.

The goal of psychoanalytic treatment therefore is to provide freedom to be curious, and to break signifies defences, such as the denial, disavowal and dissociations, that defend against fear of what one would think; that is, if the person allowed themselves the freedom to think it. From a psychoanalytical view, there are relationships between two fundamental experiences: (1) the verbal reflection and non-verbal experience; and (2) the experience that have not been reflected on, and not yet verbalised. I am in particular interested in the process of the unformulated experience, which is deeply felt and needed *space*, openness, a sense of wonder, curiosity, the sense of explicit verbal experience as it continuously emerges and constructs, which can lead to dialect between dissociation (both healthy and unhealthy), conjecture and imagination. The unconscious aspects of experience of course can be reconceptualised by interpretation of transference and countertransference in the interpersonal therapeutic relationship with continuous movement, between the therapist and patient together and other participants in the group and the kind of relatedness in which they are in. Psychoanalytic constructivism is important here as it posits that the therapist is unavoidably embedded in and unconsciously participates in the therapeutic process. The concept of dissociation connected social constructivism, hermeneutics, and other post-modern concepts and their relevance to clinical practice, indeed, the clinical consequences of viewing psychoanalysis, the unconscious, transference, countertransference, interpretation, resistance in the therapeutic process of working with patients who endured trauma. How can they reflect on their experience and put it into words, and what persists in preserving them from knowing, and what does knowing something mean? Unconscious experience, interpretation and meaning is not easily accessible to be revealed or be articulated, and can be dissociated from. It is material that has never been brought into consciousness, not material that has been ejected from it.

However, they present special problems in therapy which can be explained in terms of the psychoanalytic paradox, which refers to a treatment impasse caused by an imbrication of psychopathology and various attributes of the psychoanalytic method. The mother's attitude toward her infant child has some similarity to the low-keyed objective analytic neutrality. These patients require different modes of relating which indicate that the therapist acting as the 'listening other', unlike their lack of emotional availability as a mother. These variations in treatment are not modifications or deviations from psychoanalysis; they are rather elements of the analytic process necessary for the treatment of specific types of psychopathology. Just as each patient is unique and the transference manifests itself in a particular fashion which then causes the therapist to make certain interpretations, the variations of technique address the construction of a containing and holding environment appropriate in working with such a patient.

The development or redevelopment of a 'sense of self' – its integration, its separation, its protection and the resiliency or lack of it – begins in the early developmental process in general. This is specifically important, when looking at refugee types of traumas. It is of great consequence to look at group and grouping in relations to the concepts of enemy and ally, at both conscious narratives and unconscious. The sense of belonging and being part of a group are largely dependent on individuals' 'sense of self', and individuals' cultural outlook within the community, ethnic or national group. People tend to have a potential to see their group as privileged group, something in line with what Erikson (1950) calls 'pseudo-species'. Consequently, the enemy group as sub-human are threatening and generate reactive defences. Questions arising here for psychoanalytic group works are:

1   What is the extent and degree of defensiveness that is characteristic of conflict behaviour represents personal and emotional needs of individuals to hate an enemy in order to keep the conflicted selves together?
2   To what extent does the group's (or we can say state's) superego play a role in the individual mind of the traumatised person?
3   To what extent does the traumatised person due to war and political upheaval and human rights violations have the capacity for splitting and projecting which plays a part in how one sees and feel about the others, and how in transference and in the process of projective identification, how one can make others feel?

Chapter 9

Creating the group

The concept of the self and its relevance in group

The contribution of Winnicott (1896–1971) to the development of object relations theory is importance in working with refugees. His concepts of self (true and false) and his conceptualisation of the psyche of the child as developing in relation to a real, influential parent, and his idea of environmental impingement are meaningful perceptive. Winnicott's (1965) view on trauma for infant is by linking it with the idea of impingement, indicating that in the developmental stage, impingement occurs in the form of a parent interfering or interrupting when the infant needs to be left alone, or the parent being absent when they are needed.

Winnicott's (1947) conceptualisation of the 'holding environment' which facilitates the transition to being self-sufficient, and his idea of the 'transitional object' (Winnicott, 1951) are also useful concepts in working with refugees. His theory of normative development (Winnicott, 1958b) links with his theory on the holding environment in the early stages of life, as the holding involves both physical and psychical aspects. These may or may not lead to ego-integration, the capacity for object relating, and eventually the capacity for object usage. All of Winnicott's ideas and concepts I find to be helpful in my work with individuals and groups, and applicable to working with refugees in exile.

One of the Winnicott's (1965) important concept for clinical implications in working within the group is his model of the false self as an ego defence that arises in response to environmental demands, which he beautifully explains and validates in *Playing and Reality* (Winnicott, 1971). This concept resonates closely and is relevant to the characteristic identified in some of refugees who were adopting a false self to survive the hostile environments. It is not difficult to imagine that the external world many of a refugee may have been impinged and intruded upon, resulting in the loss of 'the sense of a continuity of being' – an existential anxiety. So, the false self is a replacement for when the true self has been impinged and, in some cases totally lost. In such cases, because of an environmental impingement, the loss of the self

DOI: 10.4324/9781003401322-10

prevents normative continuity or a real state of existence in a dangerous and dysfunctional (childhood) and violent (adulthood) environment. It is also true that if someone uses a false self, then they depend very much on complying with the external world, making it possible that they may be very lost if that familiar, although dysfunctional external world, is taken away from them. This of course always raises the question of whether refugees develop a false self because they have lost everything in their world that made up their true life; or whether they are people who have always, from childhood, developed and lived as a false self because of environmental impingements to comply with their external world. When becoming a refugee, this second group are re-traumatised by the loss of their familiar although dysfunctional external world. Or is it a leaner combination of these two possibilities? There is something about internal strength and resilience that can distinguishes people who have it from people who don't.

The nature of the false self presented by some patients mainly constructed to cover and protect the true self in dangerous situations. A self may not initially have been false at all, and the false self is a defence mechanism adopted to survive, though its function is not based on true reality of the person. This false self can manifest itself in various forms and degrees. In an attuned false self-organisation, a refugee who presents an agreeable, compliant, compliant and interpersonally polite attitude may be seeking to behave in this manner that is socially expected. By doing so the person aims to develop the tendency toward falseness which serves better acceptance in new environment and provide opportunity for interpersonal involvement with the new environment. Then again, the conditions are significantly intensified in those traumatised refugee patients who do present an intrapsychic structural vulnerability of the self, which belongs to the early developmental process and may be intensified in later life, but the new intense false self is not a result of trauma in adulthood. For some people whose personality was initially affected by external trauma, and with a secondary external trauma the self may become totally distorted. This is different from the false self that intends to hide the inner realities of the true self. Hence, if the true self flourishes in response to the good enough m/other/therapist listening and facilitating environment to mourn and grieve the losses, a refugee patient who has had a good early developmental process, although traumatised in adult life prior to becoming a refugee, with the help of a good-enough analyst, able to go back and make reparations, and in so doing develop resilience and a true self.

Some of the challenge in working with people who have been affected by external trauma is knowledge of early developmental stage that is important to know to form a group. Some people with severe forms of early trauma and personality impairment, a false self-system may consist of an organisation of various part-selves, none of which are so fully developed or integrated as to have a comprehensive personality of their own. Laing (1959) called this 'divided self'. With these types of presentation there is no single true or false self exists, but various, complex and fragmented part selves constitute the personality. The self then, may experience dissociation or splitting of its embodied and disembodied aspects of being. The sense of being is subjected to existential modalities already constitutive of its being, and the true self may be structurally deficient, hence false. This falseness is not due just to self-deception. It could be due to the lack of developmental interactions that should have formed the psychological basis of a cohesive self; I see this as the foundations of resiliency and the intra-psychic space for the living self.

It is possible that a traumatised person intrapsychic structure is so impaired, for reasons of both developmental personality formation and later external persecution, so, even the emergence of a false character organisation is deficient. This is reflective of the social environment. So, in such state of mind, there is no capacity to work to begin with. Participation for such a patient can become a basis for testing, in search of a prospect for the assessment of individual with hope of building rapport towards integration of disavowed, rejected or discarded aspects of one's personality, and for the affirmation of evolving parts. This is in line with Stolorow and Atwood's (1992) 'pre-reflective unconsciousness', Bollas's (1987) 'unthought known', and also the clinical phenomenon described by many distinguished psycho-analysts under terms such as projective identification (Bion, 1967; Rosenfeld, 1971; Lichtenstein & Rosenfeld, 1983; Joseph, 1987; Sandler, 1990; Spillius, 1992; Hinshelwood, 1983, 1994, 1999; Segal, 1973), enactment (Jacobs, 1986, 1991; McLaughlin, 1992; McDougall, 1985, 1986), basic fault (Balint, 1968), and self as an object and the other (Searles, 1959, 1965, 1986; Cassimatis, 1984).

The self and the creation of an enemy group

The first time I was contemplating of setting up group for woman who has been raped violently by the officials as the torture. War always is disturbing but seeing men use their genitals as the weapon in such an unhuman way towards the end of the twentieth century was beyond my imagination. As I acknowledged earlier, the development of a sense of self; its integration, its separation, and its protection all begin in early childhood. The concepts of enemy and ally, the sense of belonging, and being part of a community or participating in a group are largely dependent on individuals' sense of self. The individuals within ethnic or national groups sometimes tend to see themselves or their community as superior and privileged and their enemy group as inferior and subhuman. So enemies are threatening and generate reactive defences. With these types of personality formation it is important to question the foundation of such development in mind, and to find to what extent the defensiveness characteristic of conflict behaviour, representing personal and emotional needs of individuals in order to hate an enemy and to keep the conflicted selves together. What is the extent of the state's super-ego influencing the individual.

To what extent in general population does our capacity for splitting and projection take part in how we see others and feel about others, and through the process of projective identification, how we make others feel about us. I refer to a valuable prototype paradigm that Pat Barker presents in her book *Regeneration* (Barker, 1991). It is the stories of Siegfried Sassoon, Wilfred Owen and others, who were treated for shell shock at some stage in the First World War by the psychiatrist and anthropologist William Rivers at Craiglockhart hospital in Scotland.

In conclusion, when we look at what psychoanalytic ideas are helpful in working with refugees, we can see that psychoanalysis provides a model for understanding trauma and how we can deal with trauma. The centrality of unconscious processes in the psychoanalytic practice is one of the impor-tance paradigm of human mind vitally important in relation to some defence mechanisms used by people endured trauma including refugees. The notions of dissociation and inner psychic space, which are central to my work in general and in this work as a whole. Free association and dream analysis as important analytic techniques and important analytic tools are more chal-lenging in the group compared to working with individuals. Work on mourning, use of language and dialogue, and relating to others who also experienced similar or same trauma in the group dynamics can be both positive and negatives. In this context I find revisiting *Mourning and Mel-ancholia* helpful to help group participants to reflect the idea of aggression as a component of human subjectivity. The work on mourning process can go into detail of complicating reality of loss and traumatic shock and by remembering and not repeating it in symbolic and dialogic manner. In the process of converting and representing loss participants in the group some-times exemplify embodying a relation between language and silence that in some sense could have been ritualised. Mourning can also involve a process of an obsessive remembrance of all types of personal and social losses and lost other in the space of the psyche, replacing the actual absence, with an imaginary presence. This restoration of the lost-other enables the participant to mourn and become able to assess the value of the relationship and understand what has been lost in losing the other. My job and specific undertaking to perform was an ordinary mourning for the person seeking to convert loving remembrances into a memory, lessening the depression and can move on from the process of mourning to relatedness and self-definition. The idea is that the overwhelming mourning takes place is interpersonal and intersubjective relational medium. Therefore, in some stages of of the group various defences are constructed in response to any interpretations that par-ticipants find demanding and too much to cope with. Thus, ego organisation, or lack of it, which is in the service of adaptation to the environment is fragmented and a attaining with the affect of traumas. Such state of mind and withdrawal from self-generated spontaneity can leads to an increased repressing of impulses for free associations and instinctive expression, in so doing terminating the real self, starting the development of a false self. The false self is developed in response to vulnerable states of mind against the unthinkable and result to the exploitation of the true self. It may be constructed in response to the fear and an existential anxiety, which many refugees have experienced in the past and or present in the new environments due to immigration and social deprivation and economical poverty. I keep in mind that it is always possibility that the unconscious displacement of the emergent of the false self is within the conditions of the earliest object relations. In this context, the false self as a collection of behaviours, thoughts and feelings is stirred by vulnerability in the person early developmental stage of life and developed further. It is not just a result of external trauma in the adult life of a refugee; it must be rooted and interlinked to earlier trauma. So, the false self functions as defence against anxiety, fears of abandonment, and fear of death. It represents the vulnerability to amalgamate the whole self-object representations as the basis of ego function and resilience, so, the integrated and cohesive sense of the self does not exist for the person. As a result, the capacity for spontaneity, autonomy, creativity and self-sufficiency is blocked further and lost in a false self-created to survive the unresolved internal conflicts and external atrocities. In view of that mourning may not be just about the loss of the object but can also be about the loss of the self in the first place. It is about both fear of annihilation of the self and fear of the loss of the other; and in cases where the false self not totally but partly lost, there is no familiar false self exist anymore. These types of fragmented false self is the new but yet unfamiliar presentations of the person. What is specifically helpful to understand refugees' psychical pain from Klein (1935) and her temporary point of view is the clarity and emphasis on different angles of losses, the difference between the paranoid-schizoid position (that is fear for annihilation and total destruction of the self), and the depressive position (that is fear of the loss of the other). There is also unambiguousness in the loss of object and the griefs the psyche as an internal space have to experience; and distinctions of how lost the other loss is for the patient. The projective identification theory of mourning is helpful to see that the loss of a loved m/other/object can be equivalent to the disruption of the self even temporary. So if the self has not been totally fragmented, there may be a need for containing, restoring and reclaiming that part of lost self, which has not been able to go through consolatory mourning and may be projected onto the lost other. This is needed essential process of analysis for the patients reclaiming an autonomous and resilient self whether in the group or individually.

The persecutory anxiety and feeling of trepidation is frightening and even a reasonable functioning person ego may as the result be replaced superego, in such fragmented mind when due to excessive anxiety the ego has been lost.

The mourning of the lost ego and of the loved object can further creates persecutory anxiety and the ego loses its function and is gradually be populated with fear and guilt. The psyche that is populated by anxiety may present with occurrences indicating abnormality about internalising the object and inability to give or to identify a good enough object which may readily be available and present for refugees in the host environment. This is an indication of a total loss. So what we may see is the failure of the organisation of defence and the manners of functioning that is the loss of the familiar self. Winnicott (1971) notion of trauma as impingement offers a way to better understand this process and traumatised person relationship in all its complexity that are combinations of feelings of love and affection, indeed with rejections, violent and aggression. It is relevant to think of a state of mind which can be impinged further due to lack of cultural and language barriers that provides another dimensions integral to a fuller understanding of the possible effect and retraumatisations for refugees in the host country, indeed transmission of trauma to offspring. These are indications that personality development throughout life, from infancy to adulthood, occurs as the result of complex dialectical developmental dynamisms, important for the development of progressively differentiated, integrated, resilient and mature sense of self that is contingent on corroborating sustaining interpersonal relationships. Equally, the development of mature, reciprocal, and fulfilling interpersonal relationships depends on the growth of a mature characterisation of the self. Relatedness of the developmental line enables us as the analyst to observe and perceive more clearly the dialectical developmental processes of relatedness, connexion, affinity, empathy and self-definition. Below I will bring an anecdote of setting up a group, partly due to the forces of limitations exposed on a small charity financially as well of immigration matters at the time.

It was the late 1990s when I developed a timely, psychoanalytically oriented women's group for fourteen refugees, asylum seekers and destitute those whose asylum applications was rejected by home office without rights of appeal or any legal aid support. Ages of woman I decided to be less than one generation between participants (aged 25 to 45).

In the process of individual assessments process (between one to six sessions, depending on the person presentations) it was not difficult to observe psychotic symptoms. I aimed to gain insight into these woman lived experience in the process of assessments, and then with their participations in the group of similar experiences learn more. This was daunting as it was the first time of developing such group with psychoanalytic approach with refugee woman, but with support and great encouragements of my fellow trustee Josephine Klein, we thought I might make it possible. Josephine with excitements impressing on me that such approach and clinical outcome is crucial for wider professionals to better understand and work with such a traumatised and in some cases destitute people in one of the richest country in the world.

After the first initial assessments of all prospective participants and monitoring my notes it was not challenging to identify the main common presenting themes, including but not limited to:

- Anger, frustrations and agitations about the uncertainty in their lives and the feeling to rejections.
- Shame, embarrassments and inability of articulating traumatic endurance in simple terms.
- Disturbing memory and confusing visions of trauma individual has endured. These tended to be the sounds and scene manifestation of events the person experienced such as the loss of relatives, torture, rapes as the weapons of torture mass killing in the community in way. Some of the woman conveyed out of body experiences usually considered as psychosis, give details of hearing voices of the torturer, and sometimes experiencing the actual torture.

Reflecting on the nature of the kind of presenting issues I mentioned briefly, initially I was concern whether I am able to form such a group. With careful considerations I formed a clearer understanding from the context of symptoms and narratives presented in the process of assessments. I then could think it is possible to distinguish the psychosis from the flashbacks associated with post-traumatic stress (PTS). The trauma-related intrusive thoughts and images was not emerged as explained in the classic classifications of the post-traumatic stress disorder but somewhat to a certain extent to be entertain and realistic convincing perceptions of an identifiable or distinctive quality of real and apparent combined senses oppressed but it has been actual experience in the person past, though it was traumatic. Such experiences do not fit well with conventional Western psychiatric diagnostic categories that I discussed in detail in the chapter on trauma and post-traumatic stress disorder; it was rather hallucinations of complex trauma with perceptual disturbance. The patient prospective participants described their powerful feelings of fear and mistrust of people around and of professionals, while having a sever sense of a broken self. They also described the pain of loss and hunted memory of losing everything and feel the world is completely shattered. Countless of the painful feelings described by individuals were based on having no sense of future, even those participants who were waiting and was anxious for their asylum application also thinking whether they will still be life even their asylum would be granted. Numbers of the participants during the assessments reported suicide attempts and the intolerable agonising destruction of life to the level they wish to die as there is no prospects and ability to make up for the past and to focussed build a purposeful life in future.

The risks of those who exposed and entered terrifying violent scenery to respond to the needs of others who endured and affected by trauma by of crime, natural disasters, or domestic violence, or those with a history of childhood sexual abuse, we know we cannot provide psychoanalytic intervention objectively without feeling its impact. Trauma work involves a voluntary and deliberate use of ourselves as a restorative instrument of healing. As psychoanalysts, it is essential to constantly re-examine ourselves and be in touch and check our countertransference feelings that are our living response to our patient's emotional state at any given analytical moment at both conscious and unconscious level. Our empathic attunement to the patient experience of traumatic disturbances and suffering and its consequences are our greatest asset and our paramount principal liability. I will discuss in more details in a chapter on the concept of countertransference starting from the early meaning that Freud initially called provides as the neurotic transference of the analyst to the patient. Though he was not interested in the issue as important and essential issue that exist within the analysts both conscious and unconsciously and it be eliminated by the analyst self-reflections and self-control. He often pictured his technical approach in the impersonal terms of the strong regard of a surgeon (Freud, 1909) or even of a telephone receiver (Freud, 1912c) as the rule of abstinence with variety of multiplicity exists and expands. In contemporary psychoanalysis the concept of countertransference was widened beyond the neurotic aspects of the analyst (Winnicott, 1965; Heimann, 1950; Milner, 1969) and it can now refer to the whole of the analyst's affective responses and has become progressively more important methodological subject for analysts. While it is important to recognise the personal choice and agreement of contentment that comes from the privilege of containing and responding to the trauma of others, we know that trauma work is specialised work that is not without personal hazard. In the group our countertransference can be varied to one towards the group as a whole and towards individual participants within the group. So, giving attention and monitoring our countertransference feelings is vital in protecting ourselves as analysts, indeed for provision of better interventions with patients, and also provision of supervision for those in the caring profession.

Working in the group the identification of our countertransference and the group members to us as the analyst and to each other as an interactive perspective are important. There is therefore a need to provide a working model for the assessment of the group analyst's countertransference in terms of monitoring and testing manifestation, source, function, and impact and how best to be used. We also need to think about when it is appropriate ways for disclosure of countertransference to patients and how to consider of criteria for countertransference feelings to be used to benefit both patients and analyst, indeed how we can determine suitability of those feelings in particular time. As professionals we also need to be mindful and able to differentiate countertransference for vicarious traumatisation or what is known as secondary traumatic stress, burnout and compassion fatigue. How we can recognise and be accustomed to understand, acknowledge, accept and have appreciation for signs and manifestation of potential secondary vicarious traumatisation to ensure our psychological health and self-care as well as to look for guidelines for improvements.

What can be different between general group and specific trauma groups in an on-going psychoanalytic group and how does an analyst decide the participants to join the group, what should be focus in trauma group are some of important issues we need to consider carefully as protective shell prior to plan and setting up a group.

With all these in mind I start a group at the Refugee Therapy Centre and more after the first one. The groups would be open-ended and would be reviewed by the end of the summer, spring and the New Year. The size would be a minimum of 6 members and a maximum of 10, and the age would be approximately 25–40 years old. The group would not be appropriate for people with a history of self-harm, people suffering from manic depression or other serious mental health problems. We would be able to offer individual counselling better suited to their needs.

The aims and rationale for the group

- To encourage members of the group to identify the causes of depression/ stress/anxiety/panic, by ongoing assessment by an analyst, and through discussion around a set of questions about progress or lack of it every 12 weeks.
- To reduce the symptoms of depression/stress/panic and reported levels of distress in participants.
- To develop and build on existing coping strategies and to regain coping mechanisms.
- To improve the personal sense of empowerment within individuals. Members will be encouraged to have an active role within the group and work towards collective understanding of the situation presented in the group and issues arise from presentations, exchanging knowledge and skills.
- To encourage building ability for social contact and to facilitate connections with places needed.
- To encourage the members to take the initiative to continue as a self-help group, possibly providing support and supervision through a facilitator and in the long term, through training members of the group to become facilitators themselves.

My role as the group facilitator

- Seek to help members in their endeavours as above.
- Seek to create further opportunities for social contact.

- Seek to constitute further understanding of the members' experiences in their new economic, social, political and cultural context.
- Seek to encourage members to take an active role within the group towards increasingly becoming a self-help group.

Inclusion criteria

The group would be for people who experienced stress, anxiety, panic, or were diagnosed as suffering from mild to moderate depression by the referrer and as assessed by an RTC analyst. Indication that a group would be appropriate and the person has a degree of commitment to attend regularly.

Evaluation and monitoring

There is a need to evaluate the progress of the group in order to ensure that we achieve our objectives. I wanted to learn about how we could improve on the format of these types of group and whether possible to continue developing more group. Every 12 sessions we will have a review and evaluation session, asking participants views on progress or lack of it.

Supervision and consultations for the facilitator is vital to ensure the progress. It is vital for the group analyst to be able to reflect on the group dynamics and their role as a facilitator. The fortnightly or monthly, depending on the experience of the analysts involved.

Ground rules for the group

1   Confidentiality.
2   Support, value and appreciation of each other's experiences and differences.
3   Criticism should be with respect and constructive.
4   Give attention to one person at a time and be aware of your listening skills.
5   Good time keeping and regular attendance.
6   Participants not to meet or talk outside the group.

Chapter 10

Transference and countertransference in the group

In positive transference feelings the patient sees the analyst as a dependable, nurturing mother. In negative transference patient sees the analyst as non-nurturing, angry and fearful; in negative transference situations, even the most vulnerable patients will deny needing help from analyst. This can be due to fear of rejection or patients concerned to be judged by the analyst and in the group settings other participants in the group. Avoidance of personal and emotional rapport and connection with analyst and other participants presentations are patient defense mechanism that need to be addressed for reflection and explorations, so, the analyst should not be moving too quickly if patient cannot cope in that particular time. In many instances, patients settle and behave as everything the analyst does working well, we as analyst should not receive and understand this as authentic. We need to see it as the patient's pattern of behavior to be obedient and amenable. Contrast to this, some patients refuse to cooperate and challenge analyst intervention, argue and try to get into conflict either with the analyst or with others in the group. It is important for the analyst not to feeling hurt, ineffective or incompetent, and understands this as the patient transference projections. Those patients initially fails to progress in the group similar to their life or denies progress, unconsciously expressing anger at the analyst and an effort to frustrate the analyst and feel in control, therefore refuses any intervention and interpretations from the analyst.

In this way patients feel in control. This type of patient complains to analyst about suffering and feeling oneself as a destitute, colluding with a victim role. This in contrast is an unconscious way of asking the analyst do something to rescue me, if you care. By doing so, patient is blaming the analyst for problems. It is our job as analyst not to see patient as victim and keeps trying to encourage the patient to restore confidence and strengthen psychic capacity for thinking and reflecting of traumatic endurance, working toward understanding those as past experiences and learn to live here and now. With these types of intervention, patient may become angry and frustrated and to feel wrongly picked up and their pain and struggles is not recognised by analysts or other participants in the group, intending colluding

DOI: 10.4324/9781003401322-11

with victim role to engage analyst to focus on them. This is perverse ways of dealing with insecurities with hope to provide some relief from anxiety and distressing feelings. Some patient cannot have confidence in the process and may delve into paranoid state against the analyst, becoming annoyed at the analyst for no apparent reasons, but not able to verbalise feeling openly, thus fears and mistrust becomes real in the patient fantasy. I usually do not challenge this or pressurise patient to have confidence in the process prematurely, as I think this will be coming in the process and no need for critical interpretations in rush.

Here, I bring a brief vignette as an example: one of the patients in a group I was running said to me, 'I don't trust you, that is the reason I don't talk much.' I said to her, thanks for sharing this in the group. I don't see any reason that you should trust me. She was shocked and responded, 'Really?'. I said of course, you don't know me, and in all relationships, it does take time to build some lever of trust, in this case if I deserve your trust. She burst into tears for the first time (four months in the group); I kept silence, and so did other members. By the end of the session, I just said, we all have been with you and your pain. Her approach to the group from next session changed. She in the next session apologised to me and the group for being 'rude'. I said, you were not rude, you felt safe for the first time to be yourself in the group and you needed to let us know, and that was your way of telling us, no harm is done. I than asked her, if she could not have that encounter of anger and frustration with me in the group, could she opened up with her sadness as she did. She said I could not and would continue attacking you and rubbished the group. She than asked me why you did not respond to or asked me to leave? I said this is your group and my job is to walk with you in your journey and not exercise authority.

In this brief encounter I wanted to give paradigm that sometimes a patient in the process may become enraged at analyst over a certain interventions or interpretations and tries to generate grouping in the group against the analyst, if not succeed in attract grouping in the group the patient move to direct confrontations by criticising the analyst as incompetence, blaming the analyst for poor performance and lack of understanding their feeling. In such encounter it is vitally important for us as the analyst to remain calm, collected and caring to reassure patient without directly working on the inner critic and without dealing with underlying issues at that particular time.

Some patients expect analysts' admiration and act as if they are superior, with improper demeaning behaviour towards the analyst. In my view, it is best not offer appreciation, thinking it may fulfil the patient needs, neither we should challenge the patients for arrogance manner in an unsupportive way. With this type of patient's demand for attention I very briefly acknowledge the exceptional view and move on. It is helpful not to favour the particular patient in transference as well as protecting other participants of engaging with a member narcissistic wounding while indicating and acknowledging the issue, there is no need to limit the group encounter due to my feeling as the analyst and potentially the limitation of my capacity to cope with confrontations. If not careful with such encounter from some patient in the group we can enter to a primitive mechanism of defense characterised by a good and bad members, or love and hate, or healthy attachment and detachment and rejection creating splitting in the group. Such split is representative deeply in the mind of patient's psychic structure, acts as a powerful unconscious force to protect against the ego's perception and affects of intense anxiety. If as an analyst I enact creating splitting in the group, I accept that I no longer a right analyst for the group, because I become one of the patient acting out, so, there is no analyst in the room anymore. This of course will leads to destructive activities and confusion in patients in the group. Splitting is an expectable part of early developmental stage to build up ego strength and ability to tolerate inconsistent and paradoxical affects, and to amalgamate and integrate well and bad, love and hate along with the related affects and various probable and difference on a subject matter become bearable ad acceptable.

Here, I will bring another brief example of a woman I have worked with who was struggling with her inner turmoil. She finds someone in her community who seems kind, respectful, mindful and responsive to her needs. She was pleased and idealised this man and invests in him with strength, love and giving. This man for her was outstanding human shining in her eyes and she could not resist the temptation to accept anything he asked as she sees him as wonderful and extraordinary person for her. Her experience with this man was all good. As we all in the group might expect, this man could not live to the patient expectations and let down the patient's idealisation by evidence of being a human with all sort of limitation and imperfection. Patient comes to the group overwhelmed and with intense induced anxiety. She felt this man is her enemy as he attacked her honour and principles, and he used her kindness and trust on him. Patient though angry, was amenable to my gentle interpretations of her fantasied style for relationship. Having said this she starts searching for a man who in her view can be honest and love her.

The intensity of my countertransference reactions in such situations was to introject the patient frustrations. Thus, sometimes come to light throughout group encounter with a patient or more than one patient in the group whose primary mechanism of defense was splitting. This would be unexpected and occasionally fear or guilt provoking for me. I needed to have space to think and reflect how best to deal with these countertransferences in any moments before making any interpretations, whether it is best offering interpretations or more appropriate to make realignment with something I am sure I can manage. In these types of situation at particular time I was aware I need to think and reflect on my thoughts and feeling more, so, I can move away and forward from my countertransference feelings. By doing so, I could gain a clearer understanding of my own developmental history that helps to reserved, gaining access to my own affects and not projecting it to patients. Having said this, as the analyst we need to be conscious of the fact that even we know our own past histories and may have had a very good analyst and supervisors it does not mean we always can eliminate our emotional responses in relations to others, and for sure it does not mean we are always conscious of our feeling and actions, there are always unconscious elements. In view of the fact that we cannot always be conscious of our own feelings, we cannot avoid the compulsion to retreat or be protective, so, our immediate thought in such circumstances and out conviction is to find the best way. This process of focusing on going forward therapeutically hopefully do conjuring tricks to get past what at times may seem unmanageable countertransference. Not reacting our feelings being clear to us at the conscious level as an analyst we immerse ourselves in searching for unknown known.

Furthermore, when a patient in difficulty come to a melancholic mournful cry of despair or launch an attack at us verbally, we need to hold back the impulse to become overly defensive or completely withdrawal. If this level of transference–countertransference erupts we need to find ways to identifying patient perception, why and what is it in the patient's history prophesy that is leading to such eruption of affect and what is it that creates internal conflicts in us. This unknown known can of course cause anxieties engendered by the patient's attack. At the conscious level we can focus on the clinical reality of the moment which can increases our ability to be understanding, empathic and accepting, but we also need to search for our unconscious reality that created discomforts, fear and anxiety in us. An interpretation of our break-through at the later stage when we have a better understanding will surely help the patient puzzling feelings of fears and rage that was projected in transference. Usually during the beginning phase of group work as much as possible I focus on patients sharing history within the boundaries of the group and identify the painful and intolerable affects that may lead to severe depressions or destructive behaviors while simultaneously providing a safe and holding environment. This is neither an easy nor a momentarily accomplished undertaking, but a process listening, reflecting and analysing. In this stage identifying and containing affects in my view is a core factor in building an effective prosperous analytical group. More often than not, the patients endured trauma may presents lack of trust and angry outburst, when this occurs, our job as the analysts is a gentle intervention to bring comfort to that patient and the group and further build safe enough relationship within the group.

People who have endured trauma especially in early developmental stages and have deep psychological wounding sometimes in group encounter seems as if the person cannot deal with their emotions and cannot immediately begin to fathom and understand the depths of their feelings, but somewhere unconscious or subconsciously there is awareness that the group can provide some relieve. Patients may need much more time in the beginning to alter the underlying tribulations of fears and anxieties projected in transference. For patients who present anger, if the analyst addressing the problems presented, it is best for a period to give no interpretations. For example, if analyst saying: I can see you feeling frightened about being the only person in the group with your past history – patient instead of sharing can choose either total silence or get angry with analyst, feeling the analyst intention to drive 'me' away. This is what at that particular time patient with those horrific memories, fears and rejection can cope within the group. While explorations is good, at this stage of patient engagements or lack of it, it is not helpful to facilitate patient to explore more feelings and memory, contrary it can make the patient feel even more inadequate and ashamed in the group and even leads to complete psychological collapse.

As an alternative, as analysts we can demonstrate interest in listening sympathetically to the intensity of patients without any encouragement or any critical interpretations. By just being the listener it is possible to help the patient to feel better. In these cathartic instances we can provide possibility for patient better engagement in the group reaches to therapeutic relationships that can gradually address those primitive fears, cause of the patient anxiety. As analyst we constantly need to remind ourselves that working with patients suffering from past trauma we need to start with an acceptance attitude that people live in an immature psychological world that stimulates or maintains emotional vulnerabilities, and they learned to guard themselves from conflict and anxiety by splitting the world into all good and all bad. Gentle interpretive intervention can provide an erroneous sense of psychological safety and renders relationships needed to stabilise the patient in an engaging and consistent manner in the group. This is a technique of maintaining and containing and being a good enough listening m/other/analyst that can open some psychic space for angry and fearful patients to think both about their affects and behavior, the reasoning for explosion of angry feeling and attack on others. Recognition of this helps patients to identify and relate to their feeling and what they are doing. Such discovery and self-understanding of transference reactions can help the development of mature psychological structures that can facilitate the relational process in the group, leading to a world less split into good and bad with contradiction. This method of working can prevent us as analyst to draw to projective identifications with particular patients within the group.

Projective identification

Projective identification an intrapsychic and interpersonal phenomenon can surely have negative effects on the analytic relationship within the group. Projective identification can draw the analyst into various forms of enactments, more so when we are not able to gain an understanding of what is going on in the group and may jump to unnecessary early interpretation as unconscious self-protections, while actually what we are doing is acting out the patient's core fantasies and feelings. Klein (1946) sees projective identification as much of the hatred against parts of the self that is directed toward the other. This leads to a particular form of identification which establishes the prototype of an aggressive object relation. I think the projective identification is parts of ourselves and internal objects that are split off and projected into the external object, which in our fantasy we can control. It is an unconscious fantasy of love and hate feelings being submitted into the internal and external object, directed toward the ideal object to avoid separation, or it directed toward the bad object to gain control of the source of danger, it also can represents a very primitive means of communication that can lead to our countertransference stress and subsequent unreasonable compulsive neurotic interactions with our patient. This process can lead to the fantasy of reinternalising a wounded object, causing depression and fear, or reinternalising a now hostile and dangerous object, triggering persecutory anxieties.

Projective identification can be for both patient and analyst alike and can excite stimulating escape of split off part of the patient mind searching for possibility to mobilise fantasies. It is acting out process of releasing internal malevolence into the object, but by denial of connection with the fragment part of the self. This can be perceived by the analyst as straightforward and uncomplicated projection, in which the ego is responding to the patient object and a sort of relationship to that object in fantasy, but by acting out and projecting that is in reality a denial of the relationship. The intrapsychic and interpersonal communications between analyst and patient can continue in this way for some time which can be frustrating for the analyst and in the process the analyst may feel blocked therefore countertransference anxiety increases which can leads to analyst acting out and in a hastily interpret patient's unbearable projections. These types of encounters are indication how projective identification can lead to intense reactions in both patient and analyst.

In the therapeutic encounter both patient and analyst wish to eradicate confrontation and distress. In part, the patient seeks an enacting response and the analyst may get impulse to enact without processing the patient enactments. This may range from good perception and tolerance of embracing the patient with empathic words to hostile responses or silence to depriving the patient desire and the part-object submissive encounter. Here, both the analyst and patient drawn to some sort of acting out that can be very enigmatic and mysterious but subtle and gratifying. Our job as the analyst here is to try to recognise, appreciate and work with enduring projective fragmented but relevant material that is left behind or misplaced by the patient in the course of projective identification. In a psychoanalytic process, we are constantly dealing with momentarily psychic elements. So, our job is to be able to provide holding and containing environment for transformations. We need to work through certain mental dynamics within the sessions and after the sessions, continue working with the patient within the context of projective identification that at times we may be struggling.

Here, I shall bring a vignette on my struggle in one of the group in which I left feeling lost and alone after a difficult session. I felt used by patients who wanted to be in total control. I managed to stay silence in the session and later on reflections I realised I could have easily acted out on my counter-transference in a sadomasochistic manner to avoid my fearful component of the patient's internal object relations.

I have been working with this group just over a year on a weekly basis. Prior to forming the group, I met each individual for the group around six sessions. I needed to ensure not having too many manic and psychotic char-acteristics in the group, but one I think is helpful. One of the potential can-didates during the assessments process presented herself as positive and full of love for others, for freedom and justice, but avoided talking about herself and her personal life and any of her relationships directly. Her focus was strongly on her being political. She avoids all my questions about her as a person. In one of the sessions I commented on the fact that she was cautious of telling me who she is as a person, but keen to present herself to me as highly political and social being and I wonder if it is a matter of trust and safety, and perhaps concern about me not being on her side. She politely resist any further exploration and as usual ask me questions and said what else you want to know about me, I am telling you everything I can but don't know much about you. We managed to pass the process of assessment and I decided to invite her to the group of women I was setting up. To my surprise she accepted. A few months into the group, she was mainly focusing on political and social issues and on occasions that she will be challenged by other group members in gentle and respectful manner, she would not come to the next or few following sessions without calling to cancel. She would not respond to my letter either, but would come back to the group as and when she wished. She was of course always having reasons to present why she couldn't attend the group and she meant to call etc. In one of the sessions, she come after missing three weeks, she seemed perplexingly awkward and uncomfortable. After explosive political preach of gender issues, she said she is very angry with her husband and had to call the police when they had big arguments a few days back. Police removed the man from the house, and after a week her children also left her to stay with their father. She then said she feels insecure in her own home and seriously concern about her children especially her daughter. This was surprising for all the group members. People in the group were supporting to her. I congratulated her in trusting to be herself in the group and gently said, her husband behavior must be quite shocking for her. She, for the first time burst to tears. After a few moments she said, his behavior was not shocking to her at all as it was not something new, but her own strength of calling the police was out of her usual character and she own this to me and the group. She could not understand why she could not trust the group. She said partly she know that she was concerned that I or participants in group may be questioning her and she didn't know what to say. One member of the group asked her if she knows now. Another member asked since when her husband shown anger and so on. I gently remind the participants in the group, much of questions in our mind surely come from the place of care, but we hear about it when time is good for that individual to share and it is good if we can stay with that. I then faced her and said we are with you. She burst to tears again. She shared with the group that her husband was violent and abusing her since the first night of their marriage but always blamed her to making him angry. She kept silence because she was embarrassed to talk even to her sister that she feels that they are very closed. As we were close to the end of the session, I was concerned, so, I suggested we could allocate some time to her next week for her to explore her experiences if she wanted too in an atmosphere of trust, that is, if everyone agreed. All members said yes. This was a good session for her and I was pleased as I thought my intervention was appropriate. Next session she first thanks everyone in the group for understanding and for allowing her time for further explorations this week and she was especially appreciative to me of ending the sessions in a must 'artistic' way that she didn't leave in tears and deep emotional pain. She felt understood and now she can see how therapy is working and how a good therapist is important. She felt like a baby with a great mother she never had and she now can see what it meant to feel safe, understood and having space. She goes on apologising for being rude and dismissive to me etc. at this point I thought she is so terrified to use the space she was offered and unconsciously passing the time, not to talk about her pains. I just said, thank you for giving me confidence that I do my work well, let's focus on you, and for the first time she listened without any challenge or argument.

In this therapeutic encounter this particular patient within the group could turn her distorted passive aggressions that she has been denying before to an active relational connection by the use of projective identification. She projected the parts of herself that she was ashamed and scared of being herself, object to her husband for the abuse and never told anyone, even close family member (her sister), managed to interject her experiences in the group and other participants' ability to feel safe into a rational representation and in that session projected her change onto group interpersonally. These become possible for her due to the sharing of her experiences of domestic violence that was addressed in the group by other members empathically. She was then said she was so afraid of sharing that part of her life and being rejected, attacked and humiliated by group and perceived as a pathetic weak and stupid woman, but focusing on the political activity and injustices both helped her to present her anger and also being admired and respected for being intelligent and doing so much good for a better world she deeply desired. All group members respond to her with respectful consideration and compassion. To our surprise another participants also could share that her husband who was executed many years ego in her country was violent as well, but she could not talk about it as he is not life and he was a well known very respectful person in her community.

This vignette of the group encounter was a clear example how harmony, respect, unity from relational perspective is possible to be achieved in trans-ference – countertransference even when we are working with severely trau-matised vulnerable if as an analyst, we can recognise people resistant and inflexibility due to vulnerability and fears due to the trauma they have endured and interjected as the bad internalised object.

I find Bion's and Rosenfeld's ideas of containment-contained and projec-tive identifications combine with Winicott's theory of containing and facil-itating environment great tools in working in the group. I learn from these that projective identification is a type of defence and a psychic process that is both concurrently and separately communicating primitive kind of object relationship, and a pathway for change. As a defence, projective identification unconsciously work to assist patients who still cannot deal with the after-math of traumatic events to create a sense of psychological distance from terrifying and fear-provoking aspects of the self as the mode of communica-tion. So, in a sense projective identification is a process by which feelings harmonising the incompatible part of one's own are bring on in another person, thereby creating a sense of being understood by or of being at one with other. This process is an integral parts of object relationship theory as represent and signify a way of being with and relating to a partially separate object. This is a channel for emotional and in many ways psychosomatic change. It is a process by which feelings like individuals struggling with are psychologically processed by another person and made available for re-internalisation come into being in a transformed shape. Functions of projec-tive identification develop and progress further in the context of the child-hood early developmental stage attempts to comprehend, systematise, and take charge of one's internal and external experience and to communicate with environment.

In the vignette above, patient used projective identification as defense to protect herself from the fear of being exposed, she feared to communicate her emotional turmoil with the group in corresponding with early intrapsychic connections. Another member of the group after this process also started feeling much more comfortable to connect with her past. She started saying now she can see this group is fit for her. She presented a paranoid state of the mind outside the group and now could express her feeling to have those feeling with the group too, believing she needed. For the first time in the group she disclosed that she was forced by her child social worker to come to therapy, she was very angry with that woman and hated her, but her view changed now and she is thankful to her. She said she felt so scared they take her child from her, and that was the only reason she agreed to come to the group but she could not trust the process as she see it as part of the whole system of control and she didn't want to say something that I as her therapist report to the authority. This woman's critical superego haunted her, causing her to be weak and she through projective identification, attempted to releases the punitive internalised part of herself into other objects for relief. Then she would feel attacked and controlled by those punitive objects. In one of the sessions, I said she wish me to show her the way out of her anxieties and confusions, but in her mind, I swiftly hurriedly change into an awful bad person who would abandon her and may attack her, humiliating and embarrass her in the group. She was responsive to my interpretation and group member silence at that moment helped her to relax and we could as group discuss her feelings and thoughts more. This process was satisfying transformation in this particular group. Another patient's use of projective identification take place in the same session where she felt victimised mistreated and useless. She said this is what the system doing to her as an asylum seeker. They don't understand that no one wish to leave their familiar environments unless their life is in danger. She assert that officials were making immeasurable finger pointing that makes me to feel this way, everything I say, they questioning it as they are interviewing a criminal. They try to catch me to make mistakes to accuse me of being dishonest. Sometimes I feel ashamed and unable to know what to say. She at this point become tearful and take the rest, but she opened another avenue from the personal to societal experiences. I needed to find a right way to connect those experiences that members shared so generously. I felt all the group members in that series of sessions were trying to use projective identification as I presented a few sessions before to discharge their anger, shame and humiliations not to each other but into me as considering me as part of the system. By doing so, they try to distracting themselves from unmanageable anxiety while unconsciously trusted me enough to let me in to their mind populated by the trauma they have endured and until now they could not face it. I considered this as a great move in the group and I usually only would say, well we had a good session today. I felt difficult disclosures need positive acknowledgements. I thought this is important as in different ways all participants were making effort to give it a go and share feeling of shame and humiliations within the group, though sometimes would projected to me with a hope that I may know how the person feels, even on occasions seeing me for sure one in the system.

With these brief vignettes I aim to address what was concurrently taking place within the group and each individual sense of the self and object differentiation or union of the intrapsychic and interpersonal aspects of projective identification. Patients were discharging undesirable aspects of themselves into me as an object they now felt safe enough in transference. They wished to abandon the deadly poisonous spiteful parts of the internal objects by projecting them out to me with hope that I can contain them. My countertransference turned into feeling a little anxious to be put in that position in patients mind and the fact if in their mind I do not fulfill the expectations I will be perceived that I was being made out to be the persecutory person. As the analyst my countertransference was part of the analytic relationship and patients' development in the group. This emotion and fear of failure in my analytic work provoked in me I find to be valuable analytical tool to be used to gain insight into transference – countertransference unconscious conflicts and defences, and try to think what is my own anxiety or insecurity and what is I am introjection from patients projections. Then, with careful interpretations we could work through making positive changes in the patient's ego and strengthening a better sense of self so they can see me as a human being, and able to build therapeutic relationship in the analytic situation. I persistently were focusing and monitoring my countertransference emotions that particularly aroused from patients thinking for right interpretations significance to group process. As a result, by and large I wouldn't act out on my part to patients' projections.

As a psychoanalyst I see countertransference to be analytic tools for self-knowledge aiding to maintain the model of therapeutic objectivity, it is important to therapeutic interventions and full participations in the patient-analyst dyad. My reactions to the patient are shaped by the patient's behaviour any given time in the treatments of which must be shaped by my behaviour and interpretations of some of previous process in the treatments. So, I as the analyst is responsible for withstanding the failure of patients' functions within our therapeutic relationship. My source of observation and reflections for patients and I will bring knowledge and understanding of the patient character and temperament towards making progress. The work with transference – countertransference usefulness in therapeutic process may means different to different analysts based on their school of thoughts and their approach as well as their own psychological outlook. My approach is intercultural psychoanalytic therapy. One of my main focus is on patient and my similarity and differences and openly address differences with patients from outset. This in my experience for almost four decades always created interest in patient engagement. It is important to know that countertransference almost always can be identified and comprehended in response and in relation to transference, but, occasionally can esteem from our own unresolved issue in respond to patient. Generally speaking, in psychoanalysis transference refers to the process by which the unconscious desires become actual and are projected onto the analyst by patient. This is happening in the process of therapeutic encounters and it is a repetition of infantile prototypes that are lived out with a deep feeling of reality. Laplanche and Pontalis (1973) understanding of transference is incongruity, resistance and repetition of the past. This incongruity relates to the analysis of here and now within therapeutic dyad and behavior of the patient towards the analyst which will provide opportunity within therapeutic relationship as a base and core for interpretations and insights.

Transference is a re-emergence of the patient's past experiences that unconsciously projected onto the analyst. If we accept the process of transference affects both patient and analyst as participants in the therapeutic relationship, it makes perfect sense to understand that the analyst is not free from the unconscious and if not careful may react to the patient inappropriately. Within this understanding it is not difficult to see that countertransference can present in any caring professional relationship and not just in analytic process, and influences professional encounters as the care giver to those in need of care. So, it is vital to always monitor and evaluate our own experience by working through unconscious. Doing so, we help ourselves to a greater understanding of ourselves and our patients, indeed a good therapeutic relationship.

Bibliography

Aberbach, D. (1989). *Surviving Trauma: Loss, Literature, & Psychoanalysis.* New Haven, CT: Yale University Press.

Abraham, K. (1913). A constitutional basis of locomotor anxiety. In K. Abraham, *Selected Papers*, pp. 235–243. New York: Basic Books.

Ahumada, J.L. (1994). What is a clinical fact? Clinical psychoanalysis as inductive method. *Int. J. Psycho-Anal.*, 75, 949–962.

Ahumada, J.L. (1997). Psychoanalysis, science and the seductive theory of Karl Popper' *Int. J. Psychoa-Anal.*, 78, 1105–1118.

Alayarian, A. (2007). *Resilience, Suffering and Creativity: The Work of the Refugee Therapy Centre.* London: Karnac Books.

Alayarian, A. (2008). *Consequences of Denial: The Armenian Genocide.* London: Karnac Books.

Alayarian, A. (2011). *Trauma, Torture and Dissociation: A Psychoanalytic View.* London: Karnac Books.

Alayarian, A. (2015). *Handbook of Working with Children, Trauma, and Resilience.* London: Karnac Books.

Alvarez. A, (1992). *Live Company: Psychoanalytic Psychotherapy with Autistic, Borderline, Deprived and Abused Children.* London: Routledge.

American Psychiatric Association. (1994). *Diagnostic and Statistical Manual of Mental Disorders*, 4th edition [*DSM-IV*]. Washington, DC: American Psychiatric Association.

American Psychiatric Association. (2000). *Diagnostic and Statistical Manual of Mental Disorders*, 4th edition, revised [*DSM-IV-TR*]. Washington, DC: American Psychiatric Association.

American Psychiatric Association. (2013). *Diagnostic and Statistical Manual of Mental Disorders*, 5th edition [*DSM-5*]. Washington, DC: American Psychiatric Association.

Anderson, R. (ed.) (1992). *A theory of thinking: Clinical Lectures on Klein and Bion.* London: Tavistock.

Andrews, G., Stewart, G., Morris-Yates, A., & Holt, P. (1990). Evidence for a general neurotic syndrome. *British Journal of Psychiatry*, 157, 6–12.

Atwood, G.E., & Stolorow, R.D. (1984). *Structures of Subjectivity: Explorations in Psychoanalytic Phenomenology*, New York: Analytic Press.

Bailey, S.D. (1963). *The United Nations, A Short Political Guide.* London: Pall Mall Press.

Balint, M. (1959). *Thrills and Repression*. Richmond: Hogarth Press.

Balint, M. (1968). *The Basic Fault*. London: Tavistock Publications.

Barker, P. (1991). *Regeneration*. London: Viking.

Barlow, D.H. (1988). *Anxiety and Its Disorders*. New York: Guilford Press.

Barrett, W.C. (1939). Penis envy and urinary control; pregnancy fantasies and con-stipation: Episodes in the life of a little girl. *Psychoanalytic Quarterly*, 8, 211–218.

Beck, A.T. (1976). *Cognitive Therapy and the Emotional Disorders*. New York.

Beck, A.T. (1983). Cognitive therapy of depression: New perspectives. In P.J. Clayton & J.E. Barrett (eds), *Treatment of Depression: Old Controversies and New Approaches*, pp. 265–290. New York: Raven.

Beck, A.T., Laude, R., & Bohner, M. (1974). Ideational components of anxiety neurosis. *Archives of General Psychiatry*, 31, 319–325.

Beck, A.T., & Steer, R.A. (1993). *Beck Anxiety Inventory Manual*. San Antonio, TX:

Bion, W.R. (1957). Differentiation of the psychotic from non-psychotic personalities. *The International Journal of Psychoanalysis*, 38, 266–275.

Bion, W.R. (1959). Attacks on linking. *International Journal of Psychoanalysis*, 40, 308–315.

Bion, W.R. (1962a). A theory of thinking. *International Journal of Psycho-Analysis*, 43, 306–310.

Bion, W.R. (1962b). The psycho-analytic study of thinking. *International Journal of Psycho-Analysis*, 43, 306–310.

Bion, W.R. (1962c). *Learning from Experience*. London: Heinemann.

Bion, W.R. (1965). *Transformations*. London: William Heinemann.

Bion, W.R. (1967). *Second Thoughts*. London: William Heinemann.

Blake, D.D., *et al.* (1995). The Development of a Clinician-Administered PTSD Scale. *Journal of Traumatic Stress*, 8, 75–90.

Blatt, S.J. (1974). Levels of object representation in anaclitic and introjective depression. *Psychoanalytic Study of the Child*, 29, 107–157.

Blum, H.P. (1980). The value of reconstruction in adult psychoanalysis. *The International Journal of Psychoanalysis*, 61, 39–52.

Blum, H. (1994). *Reconstruction in Psychoanalysis: Childhood Revisited and Recreated*. New York: International University Press.

Blum, H. (2000). The reconstruction of reminiscence. *Journal of American Psychoanalytic Association*, 47, 1125–1144.

Blum, R.W., *et al.* (2003). Adolescent Health in the Caribbean Risk and Protective Factors. *American Journal of Public Health*, 93, 456–460.

Bollas, C. (1987). *The Shadow of the Object*. New York: Columbia University Press.

Bollas, C. (1989). *Forces of Destiny, Psychoanalysis and Human Idiom*. London: Free Association Books.

Bowlby, J. (1969). *Attachment and Loss*, vol. 1. New York: Basic Books.

Bowlby, J. (1973). *Attachment and Loss*, vol. 2. New York: Basic Books.

Bowlby, J. (1980). *Attachment and Loss*, vol. 3. New York: Basic Books.

Bowlby, J. (1988). *A Secure Base: Clinical Applications of Attachment Theory*. London: Routledge & Kegan Paul.

Braithwaite, R.B. (1953). *Scientific Explanation: A Study of the Function of Theory, Probability and Law in Science*. Cambridge: Cambridge University Press.

Breier, A., Charney, D.S., & Heninger, G.R. (1984). Major depression in patients with agoraphobia and panic disorder. *Archives of General Psychiatry*, 41, 1129–1135.

Breuer, J., & Freud, S. (1895). Studies on hysteria. In *The Standard Edition of the Complete Psychological Works of Sigmund Freud* (ed. J. Strachey). Richmond: Hogarth Press.

Burr, V. (2003). *Social constructionism*, 2nd edition. Abingdon: Routledge.

Busch, F.N., *et al.* (1991). Neurophysiological, cognitive-behavioral, and psychoanalytic approaches to panic disorder: Toward an integration. *Psychoanalytic Inquiry*, 11, 316–332.

Cassimatis, E.G. (1984). The 'false self': Existential and therapeutic issues. *International Review of Psycho-Analysis*, 11(1), 69–77.

Chambless, D.L., Caputo, G.C., Bright, P., & Gallagher, R. (1984). Assessment of fear of fear in agoraphobics: the body sensations questionnaire and the agoraphobic cognitions questionnaire. *Journal of Consulting and Clinical Psychology Review*, 4, 431–457.

Coltart, N. (1988). *How to Survive as a Psychotherapist*. London: Sheldon.

Compton, A. (1972). A study of the psychoanalytic theory of anxiety: I. The development of Freud's theory of anxiety. *Journal of the American Psychoanalytic Association*, 20, 341–394.

Compton, A. (1980). A study of the psychoanalytic theory of anxiety: III. A preliminary formulation of the anxiety response. *Journal of the American Psychoanalytic Association*, 28, 739–773.

Cooper, A.M. (1993). Discussion: On empirical research. *Journal of the American Psychoanalytic Association*, 41, 381–391.

Craske, M. (1991). Phobic fear and panic attacks: The same emotional states triggered by different cues? *Clinical Psychology Review*, 11, 599–620.

Creamer, M.C., Burgess, P., & McFarlane, C.A. (2001). Post-traumatic stress disorder: findings from the Australian National Survey of Mental Health and Well-being. *Psychological Medicine*, 31(7), 1237–1247.

Dahl, H. (1979). *Word Frequencies of Spoken English*. Essex, CT: Verbatim Press.

Darwin, C., (1859). *On the Origin of Species*, London: John Murray.

Davidson, J.R.T. (1996). *Davidson Trauma Scale*. North Tonawanda, NY: Multi-Health Systems.

DiNardo, P.A., O'Brien, G.T., Barlow, D.H., Waddell, M.T., & Blanchard, E.B. (1983). Reliability of DSM-III anxiety disorder categories using a new structured interview. *Archives of General Psychiatry*, 40, 1070–1074.

Eaton, W.W., & Keyl, P.M. (1990). Risk factors for the onset of agoraphobia in a prospective, population based study. *Archives of General Psychiatry*, 47, 819–824.

Edelson, M. (1984). *Hypothesis and Evidence in Psychoanalysis*. Chicago, IL: University of Chicago Press.

Elliott, A., & Frosh, S. (1995). *Psychoanalysis in Contexts: Paths between Theory and Modern Culture*. London: Routledge.

Erikson, E.H. (1950). *Childhood and Society*, 2nd edition. New York: Norton.

Erikson, E.H. (1964). *Insight and Responsibility Lectures on the Ethical Implications of Psychoanalytic Insight*. New York: Norton.

Everly, G.S., & Mitchell, J.T. (2000). The debriefing 'controversy' and crisis intervention: A review of the lexical and substantive issues. *International Journal of Emergency Mental Health*, 2, 211–225.

Ezriel, H. (1950). A psycho-analytic approach to the treatment of patients in groups. *Journal of Mental Science*, 96, 774–779.

Ezriel, H. (1956). Experimentation within the psycho-analytic session. *British Journal for the Philosophy of Science*, 7, 29–48.

Fairbairn, W.R.D. (1929a). Is the superego repressed? In D.E. Scharff & E.F. Birtles (eds), *From Instinct to Self: Selected Papers of W. R. D. Fairbairn*, vol. 1. New York: Jason Aronson.

Fairbairn, W.R.D. (1929b). Repression and dissociation. In D.E. Scharff & E.F. Birtles (eds), *From Instinct to Self: Selected Papers of W. R. D. Fairbairn*, vol. 2. New York: Jason Aronson.

Fairbairn, W.R.D. (1954). Observations on the nature of hysterical states. *British Journal of Medical Psychology*, 27, 105–125.

Figlio, K. (1982). How does illness mediate social relations? Workmen's compensation and medical-legal practices, 1890–1940. In A. Treacher & P. Wright (eds), *The Problem of Medical Knowledge: Examining the Social Construction of Medicine*.

Foa, E.B., Davidson, J. R. T., Frances, A., & Ross, R. (1999). Expert consensus treatment guidelines for posttraumatic stress disorder. *Journal of Clinical Psychiatry*, 60, 69–76.

Foa, E.B., Hearst-Ikeda, D., & Perry, K.J. (1995). Evaluation of a brief cognitve-behavioral program for the prevention of chronic PTSD in recent assault victims. *Journal of Consulting and Clinical Psychology*, 63, 948–955.

Foa, E.B., Kozak, M.J., Salkovskis, P.M., Coles, M.E., & Amir, N. (1998). The validation of a new obsessive-compulsive disorder scale: The Obsessive-Compulsive Inventory. *Psychological Assessment*, 10, 206–214.

Foa, E.B., McLean, C. P., Zang, Y., Zong, J., Rauch, S., Porter, K., & Kauffman, B. (2016). Psychometric properties of the Posttraumatic Stress Disorder Symptoms Scale Interview for DSM-5 (PSSI-5). *Psychological Assessment*, 28, 1159–1165.

Follette, W.C. (1996). Introduction to the special section on the development of theoretically coherent alternatives to the DSM system. *Journal of Consulting Clinical Psychology*, 64, 1117–1119.

Fonagy, P. (1999). Evidenced based medicine and its justifications. In M. Leuzinger-Bohleber & M. Target (eds), *Outcomes of Psychoanalytic Treatment*. London: Whurr.

Fonagy, P., & Target, M. (1996). Playing with reality: I. Theory of mind and the normal development of psychic reality. *The International Journal of Psychoanalysis*, 77(2), 217–233.

Fonagy, P., & Target, M. (1997). Attachment and reflective function: Their role in self-organization. *Development and Psychopathology*, 9(4), 679–700.

Foulkes, S. H. (1968). On interpretation in group analysis. *International Journal of Group Psychotherapy*, 18, 432–434.

Franz, C.E., & White, K.M. (1985). Individuation and attachment in personality development: Extending Erikson's theory. *Journal of Personality*, 53, 224–256.

Freud, S. (1886a). Observation severe case of hemi-anaesthesia in hysterical male. In *The Standard Edition of the Complete Psychological Works of Sigmund Freud* (ed. J. Strachey) [hereafter '*S.E.*'], vol. 1, pp. 23–34. Richmond: Hogarth Press.

Freud, S. (1886b). Preface: Charcot's 'Lectures on diseases of nervous system'. *S.E.*, vol. 1, pp. 17–22. Richmond: Hogarth Press.

Freud, S. (1892a). A case of successful treatment by hypnotism. *S.E.*, vol. 1, pp. 115–128. Richmond: Hogarth Press.

Freud, S. (1892b). Preface and footnotes: translation Charcot's 'Tuesday lectures'. *S. E.*, vol. 1, pp. 129–146. Richmond: Hogarth Press.

Freud, S. (1893a). A comparative study of organic and hysterical motor paralyses. *S. E.*, vol. 1, pp. 155–172. Richmond: Hogarth Press.

Freud, S. (1893b). On the psychical mechanism of hysterical phenomena: A lecture. *S. E.*, vol. 3, pp. 27–39. Richmond: Hogarth Press.

Freud, S. (1894). The neuro-psychoses of defence. *S. E.*, vol. 3, pp. 45–61. Richmond: Hogarth Press.

Freud, S. (1895a). A reply to criticisms of my paper on anxiety neurosis. *S. E.*, vol. 3, pp. 121–139. Richmond: Hogarth Press.

Freud, S. (1895b). Detaching syndrome of anxiety neurosis from neurasthenia. *S. E.*, vol. 3, pp. 87–115. Richmond: Hogarth Press.

Freud, S. (1896a). Further remarks on the neuro-psychoses of defence. *S. E.*, vol. 3, pp. 162–185. Richmond: Hogarth Press.

Freud, S. (1896b). The etiology of hysteria. *S. E.*, vol. 3. Richmond: Hogarth Press.

Freud, S. (1898a). Sexuality in the aetiology of the neuroses. *S. E.*, vol. 3, pp. 263–285. Richmond: Hogarth Press.

Freud, S. (1898b). The psychical mechanism of forgetfulness. *S. E.*, vol. 3, pp. 289–297. Richmond: Hogarth Press.

Freud, S. (1900a). The interpretation of dreams, part I. *S. E.*, vol. 4, pp. 1–338. Richmond: Hogarth Press.

Freud, S. (1900b). The interpretation of dreams, part II. *S. E.*, vol. 5, pp. 339–625. Richmond: Hogarth Press.

Freud, S. (1901). The psychopathology of everyday life. *S. E.*, vol. 6, pp. 1–290. Richmond: Hogarth Press.

Freud, S. (1905a). Fragment of an analysis of a case of hysteria. *S. E.*, vol. 7. Richmond: Hogarth Press.

Freud, S. (1905b). Three essays on the theory of sexuality. *S. E.*, vol. 7. Richmond: Hogarth Press.

Freud, S. (1905c). Fragment of an analysis of a case of hysteria. *S. E.*, vol. 7, pp. 7–122. Richmond: Hogarth Press.

Freud, S. (1905d). Jokes and their relation to the unconscious. *S. E.*, vol. 8, pp. 9–236. Richmond: Hogarth Press.

Freud, S. (1906a). Obsessive actions and religious practices. *S. E.*, vol. 9, pp. 117–127. Richmond: Hogarth Press.

Freud, S. (1906b). Preface to Freud's shorter writings, 1893–1906. *S. E.*, vol. 3, pp. 1–6. Richmond: Hogarth Press.

Freud, S. (1906c). Psycho-analysis and establishment of facts in legal proceedings. *S. E.*, vol. 9, pp. 97–114. Richmond: Hogarth Press.

Freud, S. (1906d). The part played by sexuality in the aetiology of the neuroses. *S. E.*, vol. 7, pp. 271–279. Richmond: Hogarth Press.

Freud, S. (1906e). The sexual enlightenment of children. *S. E.*, vol. 9, pp. 131–139. Richmond: Hogarth Press.

Freud, S. (1909). Some general remarks on hysterical attacks. *S. E.*, vol. 9, pp. 229–234. Richmond: Hogarth Press.

Freud, S. (1910a). The origin and development of psychoanalysis. *S. E.*, vol. 11. Richmond: Hogarth Press.

Freud, S. (1910b). A special type of choice of object made by men. *S. E.*, vol. 11, pp. 165–175. Richmond: Hogarth Press.

Freud, S. (1910c). Contributions to a discussion on suicide. *S.E.*, vol. 11, pp. 231–232. Richmond: Hogarth Press.

Freud, S. (1910d). Five lectures on psycho-analysis. *S.E.*, vol. 11, pp. 9–55. Richmond: Hogarth Press.

Freud, S. (1910e). Leonardo da Vinci and a memory of his childhood. *S.E.*, vol. 11, pp. 63–137. Richmond: Hogarth Press.

Freud, S. (1910f). The antithetical meaning of primal words. *S.E.*, vol. 11, pp. 155–161. Richmond: Hogarth Press.

Freud, S. (1910g). The future prospects of psycho-analytic therapy. *S.E.*, vol. 11, pp. 141–151. Richmond: Hogarth Press.

Freud, S. (1910h). The psycho-analytic view of psychogenic disturbance of vision. *S.E.*, vol. 11, pp. 211–218. Richmond: Hogarth Press.

Freud, S. (1910i). Two instances of pathogenic phantasies revealed by patients. *S.E.*, vol. 11, pp. 236–237. Richmond: Hogarth Press.

Freud, S. (1911a). The handling of dream-interpretation in psycho-analysis. *S.E.*, vol. 12, pp. 91–96. Richmond: Hogarth Press.

Freud, S. (1911b). Psycho-analytic notes on an autobiographical account of a case of paranoia (dementia paranoides). *S.E.*, vol. 12, pp. 9–79. Richmond: Hogarth Press.

Freud, S. (1912a). A note on the unconscious in psycho-analysis. *S.E.*, vol. 12, pp. 260–266. Richmond: Hogarth Press.

Freud, S. (1912b). The dynamics of transference. *S.E.*, vol. 12, pp. 99–108. Richmond: Hogarth Press.

Freud, S. (1912c). Types of onset of neurosis. *S.E.*, vol. 12, pp. 231–238. Richmond: Hogarth Press.

Freud, S. (1913a). An evidential dream. *S.E.*, vol. 12, pp. 267–278. Richmond: Hogarth Press.

Freud, S. (1913b). Observations and examples from analytic practice. *S.E.*, vol. 13, pp. 191–198. Richmond: Hogarth Press.

Freud, S. (1913c). On beginning the treatment (technique of psycho-analysis, I). *S.E.*, vol. 13, pp. 123–144. Richmond: Hogarth Press.

Freud, S. (1913d). On psycho-analysis. *S.E.*, vol. 12, pp. 205–212. Richmond: Hogarth Press.

Freud, S. (1913e). The claims of psycho-analysis to scientific interest. *S.E.*, vol. 13, pp. 165–190. Richmond: Hogarth Press.

Freud, S. (1913f). The occurrence in dreams of material from fairy tales. *S.E.*, vol. 12, pp. 279–288. Richmond: Hogarth Press.

Freud, S. (1913g). Totem and taboo. *S.E.*, vol. 13, pp. 1–161. Richmond: Hogarth Press.

Freud, S. (1913h). The theme of the three caskets. *S.E.*, vol. 12, pp. 289–302. Richmond: Hogarth Press.

Freud, S. (1913i). Two lies told by children. *S.E.*, vol. 12, pp. 303–310. Richmond: Hogarth Press.

Freud, S. (1914a). On narcissism: an introduction. *S.E.*, vol. 14, pp. 73–102. Richmond: Hogarth Press.

Freud, S. (1914b). On the history of the psycho-analytic movement. *S.E.*, vol. 14, pp. 1–67. Richmond: Hogarth Press.

Freud, S. (1914c). Remembering, repeating and working through. *S.E.*, vol. 12, pp. 145–156. Richmond: Hogarth Press.

Freud, S. (1915a). The unconscious. *S.E.*, vol. 14, pp. 159–205. Richmond: Hogarth Press.

Freud, S. (1915b). Thoughts for the times on war and death. *S.E.*, vol. 14, pp. 273–300. Richmond: Hogarth Press.

Freud, S. (1915c). Case of paranoia running counter to the psycho-analytic theory. *S.E.*, vol. 14, pp. 261–272. Richmond: Hogarth Press.

Freud, S. (1915d). Instincts and their vicissitudes. *S.E.*, vol. 14, pp. 117–140. Richmond: Hogarth Press.

Freud, S. (1915e). Letter to Dr. Hermine von Hug-Hellmuth. *S.E.*, vol. 14, pp. 341–341. Richmond: Hogarth Press.

Freud, S. (1915f). Observations on transference-love: Technique of psycho-analysis. *S.E.*, vol. 12, pp. 159–171. Richmond: Hogarth Press.

Freud, S. (1915g). Repression. *S.E.*, vol. 14, pp. 146–158. Richmond: Hogarth Press.

Freud, S. (1916a). Introductory lectures on psycho-analysis. Parts I and II. *S.E.*, vol. 15, pp. 9–239. Richmond: Hogarth Press.

Freud, S. (1916b). On transience. *S.E.*, vol. 14, pp. 303–308. Richmond: Hogarth Press.

Freud, S. (1917a). A metapsychological supplement to the theory of dreams. *S.E.*, vol. 14, pp. 222–235. Richmond: Hogarth Press.

Freud, S. (1917b). Introductory lectures on psycho-analysis. Part III. *S.E.*, vol. 16, pp. 243–463. Richmond: Hogarth Press.

Freud, S. (1917c). Mourning and melancholia [1915]. *S.E.*, vol. 14, pp. 237–258. Richmond: Hogarth Press.

Freud, S. (1917d). On transformations of instinct as exemplified in anal erotism. *S.E.*, vol. 17, pp. 127–133. Richmond: Hogarth Press.

Freud, S. (1918a). Lines of advance in psychoanalytic therapy. *S.E.*, vol. 17, pp. 157–168. Richmond: Hogarth Press.

Freud, S. (1918b). From the history of an infantile neurosis. *S.E.*, vol. 17, pp. 7–122. Richmond: Hogarth Press.

Freud, S. (1919a). A note on psycho-analytic publications and prizes. *S.E.*, vol. 17, pp. 267–270. Richmond: Hogarth Press.

Freud, S. (1919b). Lines of advance in psycho-analytic therapy. *S.E.*, vol. 17, pp. 159–168. Richmond: Hogarth Press.

Freud, S. (1919c). Introduction to psychoanalysis and war neuroses. *S.E.*, vol. 17, pp. 205–211. Richmond: Hogarth Press.

Freud, S. (1920). Beyond the pleasure principle. *S.E.*, vol. 18, pp. 7–64. Richmond: Hogarth Press.

Freud, S. (1921). Group psychology and the analysis of the ego. *S.E.*, vol. 18, pp. 69–143. Richmond: Hogarth Press.

Freud, S. (1923a). Josef Popper-Lynkeus and the theory of dreams. *S.E.*, vol. 19, pp. 261–266. Richmond: Hogarth Press.

Freud, S. (1923b). The ego and the id. *S.E.*, vol. 19, pp. 12–66. Richmond: Hogarth Press.

Freud, S. (1924a). The economic problem of masochism. *S.E.*, vol. 19, pp. 155–170. Richmond: Hogarth Press.

Freud, S. (1924b). The loss of reality in neurosis and psychosis. *S.E.*, vol. 19, pp. 183–190. Richmond: Hogarth Press.

Freud, S. (1924c). A short account of psycho-analysis. *S.E.*, vol. 19, pp. 191–209. Richmond: Hogarth Press.

Freud, S. (1926a). Inhibitions, symptoms and anxiety. *S.E.*, vol. 20, pp. 87–157. Richmond: Hogarth Press.

Freud, S. (1926b). The question of lay analysis. *S.E.*, vol. 20, pp. 77–175. Richmond: Hogarth Press.

Freud, S. (1926c). Psycho-analysis. *S.E.*, vol. 20, pp. 263–270. Richmond: Hogarth Press.

Freud, S. (1927). The future of an illusion. *S.E.*, vol. 21, pp. 5–56. Richmond: Hogarth Press.

Freud, S. (1930). Civilization and its discontents. *S.E.*, vol. 21, pp. 57–258. Richmond: Hogarth Press.

Freud, S. (1933). New introductory lectures on psycho-analysis. *S.E.*, vol. 22, pp. 5–182. Richmond: Hogarth Press.

Freud, S. (1936). *The Problem of Anxiety*. Translation by H.A. Bunker. New York: W. W. Norton & Co.

Freud, S. (1937a). Analysis terminable and interminable. *S.E.*, vol. 23. Richmond: Hogarth Press.

Freud, S. (1937b). Anti-semitism in England. *S.E.*, vol. 23, pp. 301–301. Richmond: Hogarth Press.

Freyd, J.J. (1996). *Betrayal Trauma*. Cambridge, MA: Harvard University Press.

Fried, M. (1964). Effects of social change on mental health. *American Journal of Psychiatry*, 34, 32–47.

Friedman, H.S., & Booth-Kewley, S. (1987). The disease-prone personality: A meta-analytic view of the construct. *American Psychologist*, 42, 539–555.

Gabbard, G.O. (1995). Psychodynamic psychotherapies. In G.O. Gabbard (ed.), *Treatments of Psychiatric Disorders: The DSM-IV Edition*. Washington, DC: American Psychiatric Press.

Garland, C. (ed.). (1998). *Understanding Trauma: A Psychoanalytical Approach*. London: Tavistock.

Garmezy, N. (1970). Process and reactive schizophrenia: Some conceptions and issues. *Schizophrenia Bulletin* 2, 30–74.

Garmezy, N. (1981). Children under stress: perspectives on antecedents and correlates of vulnerability and resistance to psychopathology. In A.I. Rabin, J. Arnoff, A.M. Barclay & R.A. Zucker (eds), *Further Explorations in Personality*, pp. 196–269. New York: John Wiley and Sons.

Garmezy, N. (1991). Resiliency and vulnerability to adverse developmental outcomes associated with poverty. *American Behavioural Scientist*, 34, 416–430.

Garmezy, N. (1993). Children in poverty: Resilience despite risk. *Psychiatry*, 56, 127–136.

Garmezy, N., Masten, A.S., & Tellegen, A. (1984). The study of stress and competence in children: A building block for developmental psychopathology. *Child Development*, 55(1), 97–111.

Gelpin, E., Bonne, O., Peri, T., Brandes, D., & Shalev, A.Y. (1996). Treatment of recent trauma survivors with benzodiazepines: A prospective study. *Journal of Clinical Psychiatry*, 57, 390–394.

Goldstein, A.J., & Chambless, D.L. (1978). *A re-analysis of agoraphobia. Behaviour Therapy*, 9, 47–59.

Gordon, K. (1995). The self-concept and motivational patterns of resilient African American high school students. *Journal of Black Psychology*, 21, 239–255.

Greenacre, P. (1956). Re-evaluation of the process of working through. *The International Journal of Psychoanalysis*, 37, 439–444.

Greenacre, P. (1960). Considerations regarding the parent–infant relationship. In P. Greenacre, *Emotional Growth*, vol. 1, pp. 199–224. New York: International Universities Press.

Greenberg, J.R. & Mitchell, S.A. (1983). *Object Relations in Psychoanalytic Theory.* Cambridge, MA: Harvard University Press.

Grinburg, L. (1992). *Guilt and Depression.* London: Karnac Books.

Grotstein, J. (1978). Inner space: Its dimensions and its coordinates. *International Journal of Psychoanalysis*, 59, 55–61.

Grünbaum, A. (1976a). Ad hoc auxiliary hypotheses and falsificationism. *The British Journal for the Philosophy of Science*, 27(4), 329–362.

Grünbaum, A. (1976b). Can a theory answer more questions than one of its rivals? *The British Journal for the Philosophy of Science*, 27(1), 1–23.

Grünbaum, A. (1976c). Is the method of bold conjectures and attempted refutations justifiably the method of science? *The British Journal for the Philosophy of Science*, 27(2), 105–136.

Grünbaum, A. (1976d). Is preacceleration of particles in Dirac's electrodynamics a case of backward causation? The myth of retrocausation in classical electrodynamics. *Philosophy of Science*, 43(2), 165–201.

Grünbaum, A. (1984). *The Foundations of Psychoanalysis: A Philosophical Critique.* Berkeley, CA: University of California Press.

Heimann, P. (1950). On countertransference. *International Journal of Psychoanalysis*, 31, 81–84.

Helman. C.G. (1986). *Culture, Health, and Illness*, 2nd edition. London: Butterworth.

Herbert, J.D. & Sageman, M. (2004). 'First do no harm': Emerging guidelines for the treatment of posttraumatic reactions. In G.M. Rosen (ed.), *Posttraumatic stress disorder: Issues and controversies* (pp. 213–232). New York: Wiley.

Herman, J.L. (1992). *Trauma and Recovery: From Domestic Abuse to Political Terror.* New York: Basic Books.

Herman, J.L. (2001). *Trauma and Recovery: From Domestic Abuse to Political Terror.* London: Pandora.

Higgins, G. (1994). *Resilient Adults: Overcoming a Cruel Past.* San Francisco, CA: Jossey-Bass.

Hinshelwood, R.D. (1983). Projective identification and Marx's concept of man. *International Journal of Psychoanalysis*, 10, 221–226.

Hinshelwood, R.D. (1991a). *A Dictionary of Kleinian Thought.* London: Free Association Books.

Hinshlewood, R.D, (1991b). Psychodynamic formulation in assessment for psycho-analytic psychotherapy. In C. Mace (ed.), *The Art and Science of Assessment in Psychotherapy.* London: Routledge.

Hinshelwood, R.D. (1994a). *Clinical Klein: From Theory to Practice.* New York: Basic Books.

Hinshelwood, R.D. (1994b). Attacks on the reflective space. In V. Shermer & M. Pines (eds), *Ring of Fire: Primitive Object Relations and Affects in Group Psychotherapy*, pp. 86–106. London: Routledge.

Hinshelwood, R.D. (1997). *Therapy or Coercion.* London: Karnac.

Hinshelwood, R.D. (1999a). Countertransference. *International Journal of Psychoanalysis*, 80, 797–818.

Hinshelwood, R.D. (1999b). The difficult patient: the role of 'scientific' psychiatry in understanding patients with chronic schizophrenia or severe personality disorder. *British Journal of Psychiatry*, 174, 187–190.

Hoggett, P. (1992). *Partisans in an Uncertain World: The Psychoanalysis of Engagement*. London: Free Association Books.

Holmes, J. (1991). *Textbook of Psychotherapy in Psychiatric Practice*. Singapore: Longman.

Horney, K. (1945). *Our Inner Conflicts*. New York: Norton.

Horowitz, N., Wilner, N., & Alvarez, W. (1979). Impact of Event Scale: a measure of subjective stress. *Psychosom Med.*, 41(3), 209–218.

Isaacs, S. (1952). *Developments in Psycho-analysis*. London: Karnac Books.

Jacobs, T.J. (1986). On Countertransference Enactments. *Journal of American Psychoanalytic Assocciation*, 34, 289–307.

Jacobs, T.J. (1991). *The Use of the Self*. Madison, CT: International Universities Press.

Jacobsen, E. (ed.) (1971). *Depression: Comparative Studies of Normal, Neurotic, and Psychotic Conditions*. New York: International Universities Press.

Jacobsen, E. (1959). The comparative pharmacology of some psychotropic drugs. *Bulletin of the World Health Organization*, 21.

Janet, P. (1907). *The Major Symptoms of Hysteria*. New York: Macmillan.

Joseph, B. (1987). *Projection, Identification, and Projective Identification*. London: Karnac Books.

Kernberg, O.F. (1965). Notes on countertransferences. *Journal of the American Psychoanalytic Association*, 13(1), 38–56.

Kernberg, O.F. (1975) *Borderline Conditions and Pathological Narcissism*. New York: Jason Aronson.

Kernberg, O.F. (1976). *Object Relation Theory and Clinical Psychoanalysis*. New York: Jason Aronson.

Kernberg, O.F. (1979). Some implications of object relations theory for psycho-analytic technique. *Journal of American Psychoanalytic Association*, 27, 207–239.

Kernberg, O.F. (1983). Object relation theory and character analysis. *Journal of American Psychoanalytic Association*, 31, 247–271.

Kernberg, O.F. (1993). Discussion: Empirical research in psychoanalysis. *Journal of the American Psychoanalytic Association*, 41, 369–380.

Kernberg, O.F., et al. (1989). *Psychodynamic Psychotherapy with Borderline Patients*. New York: Basic Books.

Kessler, R.C., Sonnega, A., & Bromet, E. (1995). Posttraumatic stress disorder in the national comorbidity survey. *Archives of General Psychiatry*, 52, 1048–1060.

Kessler, R.J. (1996). Panic disorder and the retreat from meaning. *Journal of Clinical Psychoanalysis*, 5, 505–528.

Khan, M.M.R. (1974). *The Privacy of the Self*. London: Hogarth.

Klein, D.F. (1993). False suffocation alarms, spontaneous panics and related conditions: An integrated hypothesis. *Archives of General Psychiatry*, 50, 306–317.

Klein, M. (1923) The development of a child. *International Journal of Psycho-Analysis*, 4, 419–474.

Klein, M. (1928). Early stages of the Oedipus complex. In M. Klein, *Love, Guilt and Reparation and Other Works, 1921–1945*, pp. 186–198. Richmond: Hogarth Press.

Klein, M. (1929). Personification in the play of children. *International Journal of Psycho-Analysis*, 10, 193–204.

Klein, M. (1930). The importance of symbol-formation in the development of the ego. *Int. J. Psycho-Anal.*, 11, 24–39.

Klein, M. (1932). *The Psycho-Analysis of Children*. Richmond: Hogarth Press.

Klein, M. (1935). *A Contribution to the Psychogenesis of Manic-Depressive States*.

Klein, M. (1940). Mourning and its relation to manic-depressive states. *International Journal of Psycho-Analysis*, 21.

Klein, M. (1945). *The Oedipus Complex in the Light of Early Anxieties*. London: Karnac Books.

Klein, M. (1946). Notes on some schizoid mechanisms. *International Journal of Psycho-Analysis*, 16, 145–174.

Klein, M. (1952a). The origins of transference. In M. Klein, *The Writings of Melanie Klein*, vol. 3, pp. 48–56. Richmond: Hogarth Press.

Klein, M. (1952b). The mutual influences in the development of ego and id. *The Psychoanalytic Study of the Child*, 7, 51–53.

Klein, M. (1975). Envy and gratitude and other works 1946–1963. *International Psycho-Analysis Library*, 104, 1–346.

Kleinman, A., Das, V., & Lock, M. (1997). *Social suffering*. Oxford: Oxford University Press.

Klerman, G.L., Weissman, M.M., Rounsaville, B.J., & Chevron, E.S. (1984). *Interpersonal Psychotherapy of Depression*. New York: Basic Books.

Kohut, H. (1966). Forms and transformations of narcissism. *Journal of the American Psychoanalytic Association*, 14, 243–272.

Kohut, H. (1971). *The Analysis of the Self*. New York: International Universities Press.

Kohut, W. (1977). *The Restoration of the Self*. New York: International Universities Press.

Kohut, W. (1978). The disorders of the self and their treatment: An outline. *Int. J. Psycho-Anal.*, 59, 413–425.

Kohut, H., & Wolf, E.S. (1978). The disorders of the self and their treatment: An outline. *The International Journal of Psychoanalysis*, 59(4), 413–425.

Kuhn, T. (1970). *The Structure of Scientific Revolutions*, 2nd edition. Chicago, IL: University of Chicago Press.

Laing, R.D. (1959). *The Divided Self*. London: Penguin Books.

Lang, P.J. (1968). *Fear Reduction and Fear Behavior: Problems in Treating a Construct*. Washington, DC: American Psychological Association.

Laplanche, J. (1999). *Essays on Otherness*. New York: Routledge.

Laplanche, J. & Pontalis, J.-B. (1964). Fantasy and the origins of sexuality. *The International Journal of Psychoanalysis*, 49, 1–18.

Laplanche, J. & Pontalis, J.-B. (1967). *The Language of Psycho-Analysis*. London: Hogarth Press.

Laplanche, J., & Pontalis, J.B. (1973). *The Language of Psycho-Analysis*. London: Nicholson.

Lazell, E.W. (1921). The group treatment of dementia precox. *Psychoanalytic Review*, 8, 168–179.

Lichtenberg, A.J., & Lieberman, M.A. (1983). *Regular and Stochastic Motion*. New York: Springer-Verlag.

Lichtenstein, A., & Rosenfeld, L.B. (1983). Uses and misuses of gratifications research: An explication of media functions. *Communication Research*, 10(1), 97–109.

Lifton, R.J. (1988). Understanding the traumatized self: Imagery, symbolization, and transformation. In J.P. Wilson, Z. Harel & B. Kahana (eds), *Human Adaptation to Extreme Stress: From the Holocaust to Vietnam* (pp. 7–31). London: Plenum Press.

Mace, C. (1995). *The Art and Science of Assessment in Psychotherapy.* New York: Routledge.

McDougall, J. (1985). *Theaters of the Mind: Illusion and Truth on the Psychoanalytic Stage.* New York: Brunner.

McDougall, J. (1986). Identifications, neoneeds and neosexualities. *The International Journal of Psycho-Analysis*, 67.

McLaughlin, J. (1992). Clinical and theoretical aspects of enactment. *Journal of American Psychoanalitic Association*, 39, 595–614.

Melzberg. B, (1964). Mental disease among foreign-born in Canada. *American Journal of Psychiatry* 120, 34–59.

Mendelson, G. (1995). 'Compensation neurosis' revisited: Outcome studies of the effects of litigation. *Journal of Psychosomatic Research*, 39(6), 695–706.

Milner, M. (1969). *The Hands of the Living God.* Richmond: Hogarth Press.

Milrod, B. (1995). The continued usefulness of psychoanalysis in the therapeutic armamentarium for the treatment of panic disorder. *Journal of the American Psychoanalytic Association*, 43, 151–162.

Milrod, B., Busch, F., Cooper, A.M., & Shapiro, T. (1997). *A Manual of Panic-Focused Psychodynamic Psychotherapy.* Washington, DC: American Psychiatric Association.

NICE. (2018). Post-traumatic stress disorder. Retrieved from www.nice.org.uk/guidance/NG116.

Pynoos, R.S., & Eth, S. (1986). Witness to violence: The child interview. *Journal of the American Academy of Child Psychiatry*, 25(3), 306–319.

Quine, W.O. (1961). *From a Logical Point of View.* Cambridge, MA: Harvard University Press.

Racker, H. (1968). *Transference and Countertransference.* London: Karnac Books.

Riviere, J. (1952). The unconscious phantasy of an inner world reflected in examples from English literature. *Int. J. Psycho-Anal.*, 33, 160–172.

Rosenfield, H.A. (1971). A clinical approach to the psychoanalytic theory of the life and death instincts: An investigation into the aggressive aspects of narcissism. *Int. J. Psychoanal.*, 52, 169–178.

Russell, B. (1948). *Human Knowledge: its Scope and Limits.* London.

Sandler, J. (1990). On internal object relations. *Journal of the American Psychoanalytic Association*, 38, 859–880.

Sandler, J., & Rosenblatt, B. (1962). The concept of the representational world. *The Psychoanalytical Study of the Child*, 17, 128–148.

Schilder, P., & Wechsler, D. (1934). The attitudes of children toward death. *The Pedagogical Seminary and Journal of Genetic Psychology*, 45, 406–451.

Searles, H.F. (1959). The effort to drive the other person crazy. In H.F. Searles, *Collected Papers on Schizophrenia and related subjects*, pp. 521–555. New York: International Universities Press.

Searles, H.F. (1965). Review of the self as the object world. *International Journal of Psychoanalysis*, 46, 529–532.

Searles, H.F. (1986). *My Work with Borderline Patients*. Northvale, NJ: Jason Aronson.

Segal, H. (1973). *Introduction to the Work of Melanie Klein*. London: Hogarth Press.

Segal, H. (1989). Introduction. In J. Steiner (ed.), *The Oedipus Complex Today: Clinical Implications*, pp. 1–10. London: Karnac Press.

Seligman, M. (1995). *The Optimistic Child*. Boston, MA: Houghton Mifflin.

Sinason, V. (2002). *Attachment, Trauma and Multiplicity: Working With Dissociative Identity Disorder*. Hove: Brunner-Routledge.

Spillius, E.B. (1992). Clinical experiences of projective identification. In R. Anderson (ed.), *Clinical Lectures on Klein and Bion*, pp. 59–73. New York: Routledge.

Stein, M.B., *et al.* (1997). Full and partial posttraumatic stress disorder: Findings from a community survey. *American Journal of Psychiatry*, 154(8), 1114–1119.

Stein J., Gorman, J.M., Liebowitz, M.R., & Fyer, A.J., (1989). A neuroanatomical hypothesis for panic disorder. *American Journal of Psychiatry*, 146, 148–161.

Steiner, J. (1993). *Psychic Retreats: Pathological Organisations in Psychotic, Neurotic and Borderline Patients*. London: Routledge.

Stekel, W. (1939). *Technique of Analytic Psychotherapy*. London: Bodley Head.

Stern, D.N. (1985). *The Interpersonal World of the Infant: A View from Psychoanalysis and Developmental Psychology*. New York: Basic Books.

Stern, G. (1995). Anxiety and resistance to changes in self-concept. In S. Roose & R. A. Glick (eds), *Anxiety as Symptom and Signal*, pp. 105–129. Hillsdale, NJ: Analytic Press.

Stolorow, R.D., & Atwood, G.E. (1992). *Contexts of Being: The Intersubjective Foundations of Psychological Life*. Hillsdale, NJ: Analytic Press.

Stolorow, R., & Atwood, G.E. (1997). Deconstructing the myth of the neutral analyst: An alternative from intersubjective systems theory. *Psychoanalytic Quarterly*, 66(3), 431–449.

Sullivan, H.S. (1946). *The Psychiatric Interview*. New York: W.W. Norton.

Sullivan, H.S. (1953). *The Interpersonal Theory of Psychiatry*. New York: W.W. Norton.

Symington, N. (1986). *The Analytic Experience: Lecturers from the Tavistock*. London: Free Association Books.

Tolpin, M. (1971). On the beginning of a cohesive self: An application of the concept of transmuting internalization to the study of transitional object and signal anxiety. *Psychoanalytic Study of the Child*, 26, 316–354.

Tuckett, D. (1994). Developing a grounded hypothesis to understand a clinical process. *International Journal of Psychoanalysis*, 75, 1159–1180.

Tyson, P. (1988). Psychic structure formation: The complementary roles of affects, drives, object relations and conflict. *Journal of the American Psychoanalytic Association*, 36(suppl.), 73–98.

Viderman, S. (1970). *La construction de l 'espace analytique*. Paris: Denoël.

Von Wright, G.H. (1957). *The Logical Problem of Induction*, 2nd edition. Oxford: Basil Blackwell.

Von Wright, G. H. (1960). Kunskapens träd [The Tree of Knowledge]. *Historiska och Litteraturhistoriska Studier*, 35, 43–76.

Werner, E.E. (1984). Research in review. *Young Children*, 39(9), 68–72.

Werner, E.E. (1992). The children of Kauai: Resiliency and recovery in adolescence and adulthood. *Journal of Adolescent Health*, 13, 262–268.

Werner, E.E. (1993). *Risk, Resilience, and Recovery: Perspectives from the Kauai Longitudinal Study*. Cambridge: Cambridge University Press.

Werner, E.E. (1994). Overcoming the odds. *Journal of Developmental and Behavioral Pediatrics*, 15, 131–136.

Werner, E.E. (1996). How kids become resilient: Observations and cautions. *Resiliency in Action*, 1(1), 18–28.

Werner, E.E., & Smith, R.S. (1982). *Vulnerable but Invincible: A Longitudinal Study of Resilient Children and Youth*. New York: McGraw-Hill.

Werner, E., & Smith, R. (1982). *Vulnerable but Invincible: A Longitudinal Study of Resilient Children and Youth*. New York.

Werner, H. (1948). *Comparative Psychology of Mental Development*. New York: International Universities Press.

Whewell, W. (1858). *The History of Scientific Ideas*. London.

Winnicott, D.W. (1947). Hate in the counter-transference. *International Journal of Psychoanalysis*, 30, 69–74.

Winnicott, D.W. (1951). Transitional objects and transitional phenomena. *International Journal of Psycho-Analysis*, 34.

Winnicott, D.W. (1958a). *Collected Papers: Through Paediatrics to Psycho-Analysis*. London: Tavistock Publications.

Winnicott, D.W. (1958b). *The Manic Defence: Collected Papers Through Paediatrics to Psychoanalysis*. London: Karnac Books.

Winnicott, D.W. (1965). *The Maturational Processes and the Facilitating Environment: Studies in the Theory of Emotional Development*. International Universities Press.

Winnicott, D.W. (1970). Living creatively. In C. Winnicott, R. Shepherd, & M. Davis (eds), *Home Is Where We Start: Essays by a Psychoanalyst*, pp. 39–54. New York: Norton.

Winnicott, D.W. (1971). *Playing and Reality*. London: Tavistock.

Winnicott, D.W. (1975). *Through Paediatrics to Psycho-analysis*. New York: Basic Books.

World Health Organization. (1992). International statistical classification of diseases and related health problems, 10th revision. Retrieved from https://icd.who.int/browse10/2019/en.

World Health Organization. (1995). *Patient Outcome Measures in Mental Health : Report on a WHO Consensus Meeting, Stockholm, 23–24 November 1995*. Copenhagen: World Health Organization.

World Health Organization. (2022). International statistical classification of diseases and related health problems, 11th revision. Retrieved from https://icd.who.int/en.

Index